GETTING REAL STRATEGIES FOR TEENS IN NEED

I HAVE DIABETES... WHAT'S NEXT?

HENRIETTA TOTH

ROSEN PUBLISHING
NEW YORK

For my niece, Emi, and my father, Eugene

Published in 2022 by The Rosen Publishing Group, Inc.
29 East 21st Street, New York, NY 10010

First Edition

Designer: Rachel Rising
Editor: Greg Roza

Portions of this work were originally authored by Leslie Green and Pat Kelly and published as *I Have Diabetes. Now What?* All new material in this edition authored by Henrietta Toth.

Library of Congress Cataloging-in-Publication Data

Names: Toth, Henrietta.
Title: I have diabetes...what's next? / Henrietta Toth.
Description: New York : Rosen Publishing, 2022. | Series: Getting real: strategies for teens in need
Identifiers: ISBN 9781499470710 (pbk.) | ISBN 9781499470727 (library bound) | ISBN 9781499470734 (ebook)
Subjects: LCSH: Diabetes--Juvenile literature. | Diabetes in adolescence--Juvenile literature.
Classification: LCC RC660.4 T67 2022 | DDC 616.4'62--dc23

Manufactured in the United States of America

CPSIA Compliance Information: Batch #CSRYA22. For further information contact Rosen Publishing, New York, New York at 1-800-237-9932.

CONTENTS

INTRODUCTION

Diabetes is a chronic, but noncontagious disease that requires lifelong management. It occurs when the levels of glucose, or sugar, in your blood are too high. Glucose is the primary source of energy and the main fuel for the brain and is derived from food. Glucose is transported to our cells by insulin, a hormone that's produced by the pancreas. The pancreas is a small organ that sits behind the stomach. If the pancreas doesn't make enough or any insulin, then the glucose stays in the blood instead of reaching the cells to supply energy.

According to the Centers for Disease Control and Prevention (CDC), more than 34 million people, or more than 10 percent of the American population, have diabetes. Nearly 27 million Americans have been diagnosed with diabetes, while more than 7 million don't know they even have the disease. The International Diabetes Federation (IDF) reports that worldwide, about 463 million adults have diabetes and this number could rise to 700 million by 2045. More than 1.1 million children and young adults across the globe have type 1 diabetes.

There are different types of diabetes. The two most common forms are called type 1 diabetes (T1D) and type 2 diabetes (T2D). In type 1 diabetes, the pancreas doesn't make any insulin so insulin must be administered each day by a needle injection or by

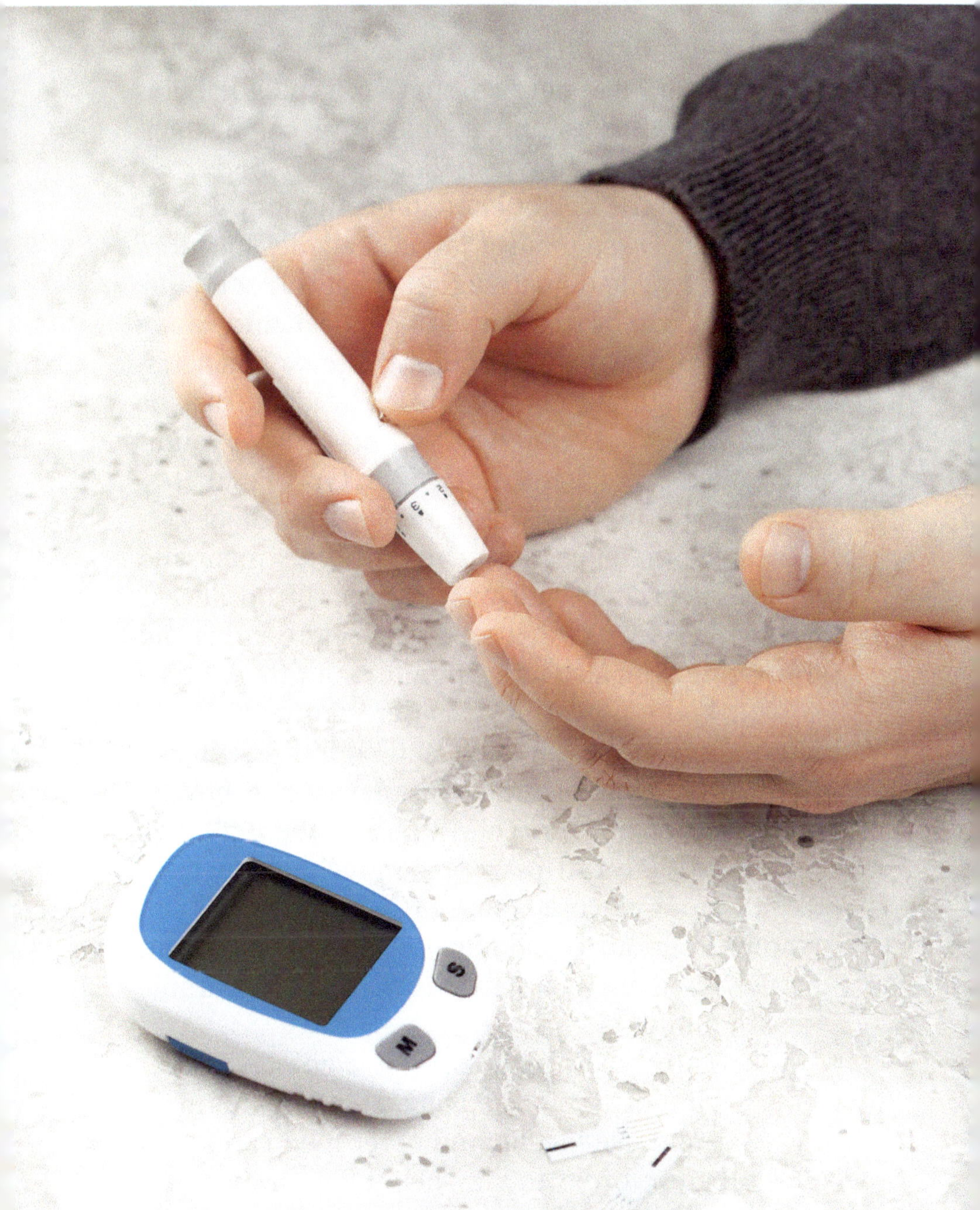

This glucose monitor uses test strips to measure the level of glucose, or sugar, in a drop of blood.

a wearable pump. This insulin helps to convert the food you eat into energy to survive. Type 1 diabetes more often affects young people, but it can be diagnosed at any age. In type 2 diabetes, the body may still make some or not enough insulin, but it can't use it properly so medication is needed. This more common type of diabetes often affects older adults, but it also can be diagnosed in children and young adults. People who have a family history of diabetes, are overweight, or are not physically active may be more prone to developing type 2 diabetes. A condition called prediabetes can lead to type 2 diabetes. Eighty-eight million Americans have prediabetes.

Having diabetes requires some adjustment and changes in lifestyle. You must test your blood glucose level several times a day, especially before eating and exercising. You also must monitor your food intake so you know how much insulin you need. You'll learn about the equipment and supplies required to measure your blood glucose levels and how to give yourself insulin. These can include a glucose monitor with test strips or a newer technology called a continuous glucose monitor (CGM) that gives you readings of your blood glucose levels. Insulin can be delivered by an injection or from a wearable insulin pump.

Currently, there's no cure for diabetes. Therefore, it's important to keep blood glucose numbers in range and use insulin and other medications as prescribed in order to stay healthy with diabetes. Uncontrolled high levels of glucose or blood sugar

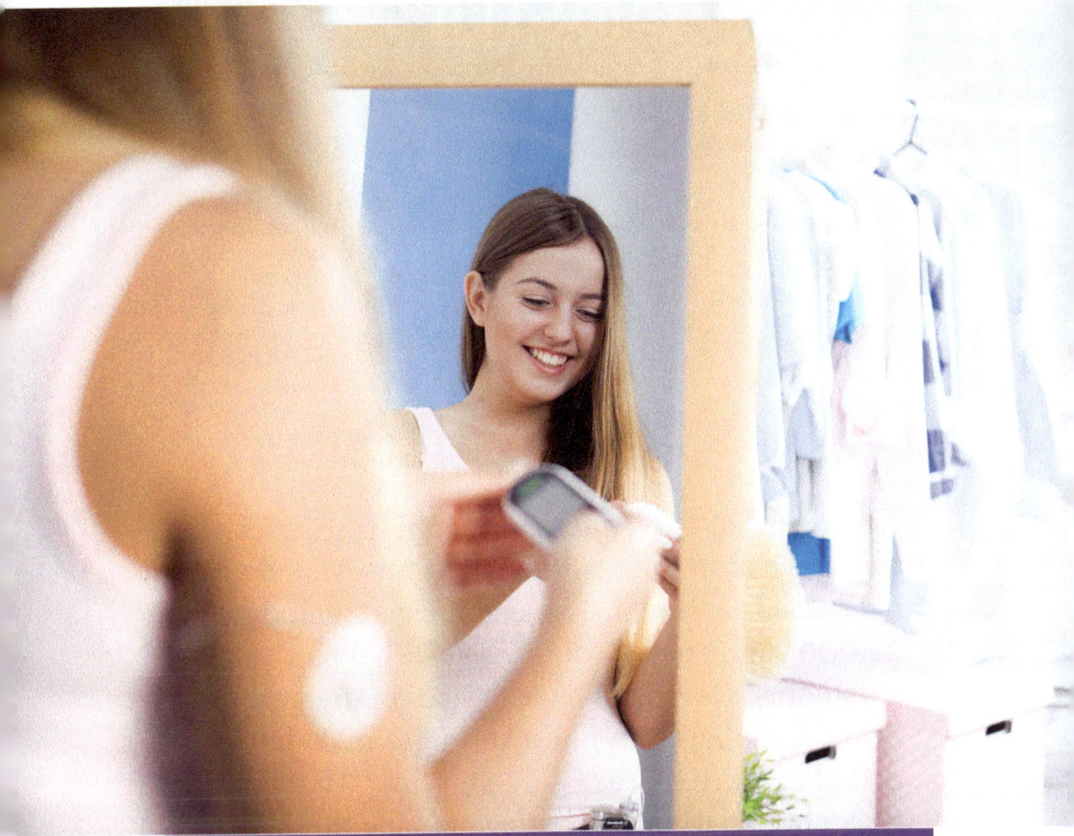

Managing diabetes may seem like a lot of work, but newer technology has made it easier than ever to monitor and regularly test your blood glucose levels.

can eventually lead to health problems, such as diseases of the eyes, heart, and kidneys, nerve damage, and even death. Diabetics can live successfully with the disease and reach their life goals through daily management of their diabetes at school, at work, on sick days, when playing sports or being physically active, and when traveling. Advances in the management of diabetes have made it easier to live with the disease, and research in better ways to manage it continues.

CHAPTER 1

DEFINING DIABETES

According to the American Diabetes Association, there are about 1.5 million new cases of diabetes diagnosed each year. These new cases include about 24,000 young people diagnosed with type 1 and type 2 diabetes. Having diabetes raises many questions: What is diabetes and how did I get it? What kinds of diabetes are there? Understanding what diabetes is can help patients to better manage their disease.

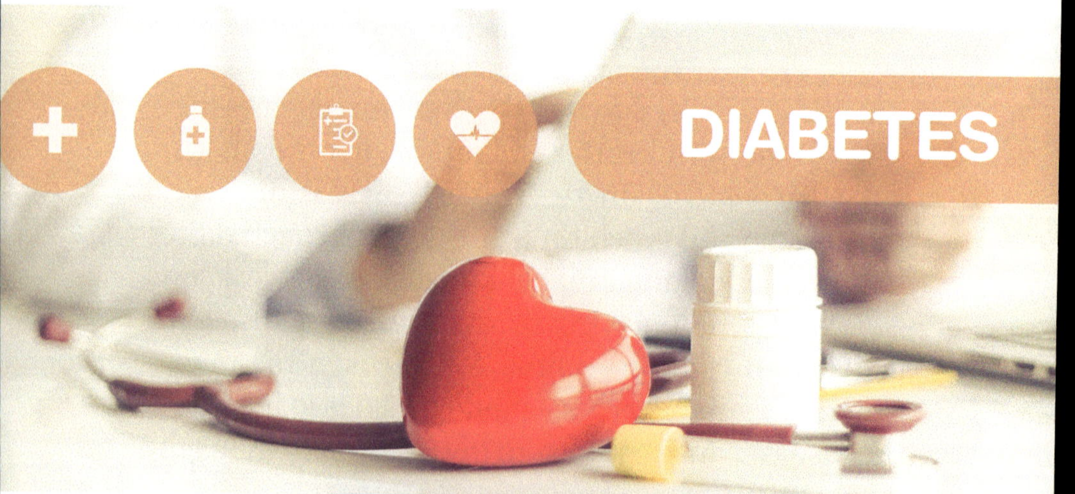

Diabetes affects many different parts of the body, including the heart.

THE CAUSES OF DIABETES

The body's immune system plays an important role in the development of diabetes. When functioning properly, the immune system protects the body from foreign substances, such as viruses and bacteria, which may enter it. However, the immune system of a person with diabetes seeks out the cells that produce insulin in the pancreas and destroys them. This causes the body to stop producing insulin either partially or completely. Without the presence of insulin in the body, diabetes develops.

Heredity also plays a role in determining who will develop diabetes, especially type 2 diabetes. A person is at a higher risk for developing diabetes if someone in his or her family has or had the disease.

THE PANCREAS

The pancreas is a long, thin organ located behind the stomach, next to the upper intestine. The pancreas is made up of two different kinds of tissue: exocrine and endocrine. The exocrine tissues make up the main part of the pancreas and produce enzymes used in digestion. The endocrine cells are scattered in clumps throughout the pancreas. These are called the islets of Langerhans. These islets are made of three different types of cells and each produce a different hormone used in the body. The alpha cells secrete glucagon, the beta cells produce the protein insulin, and the delta cells produce the hormone somatostatin.

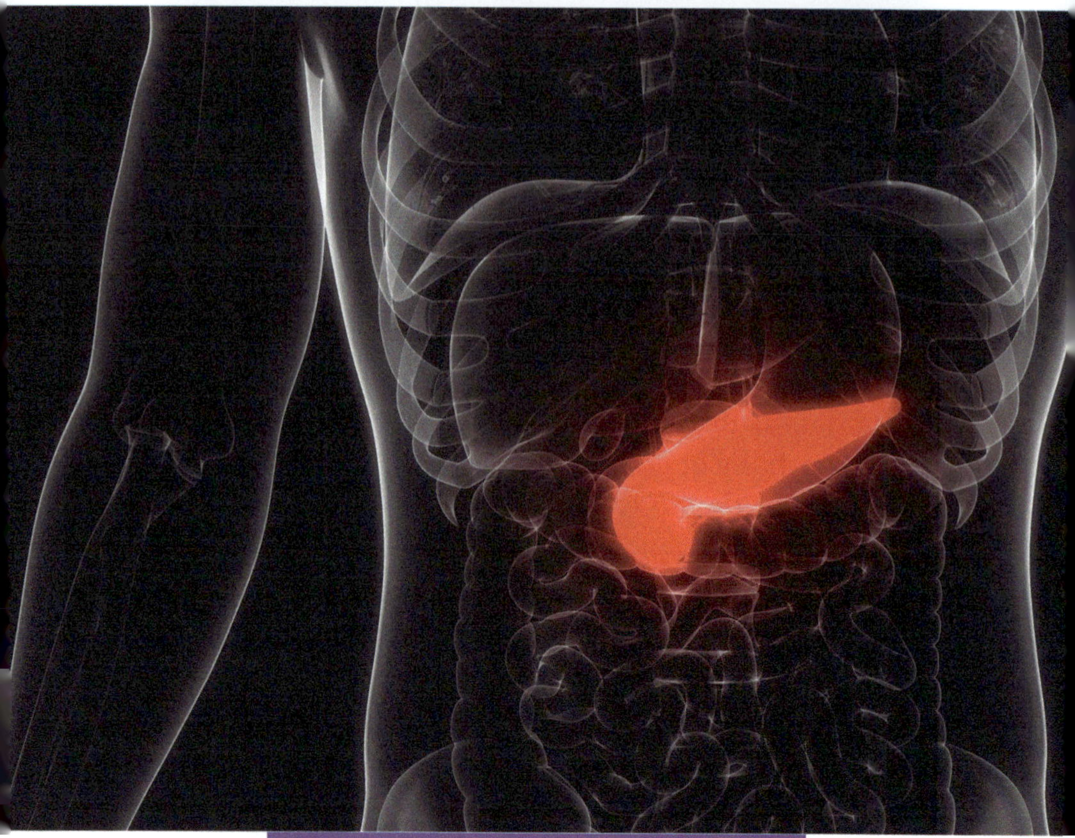

The pancreas, shown here in red, is located behind the stomach. It is about the same size as your hand.

The first two, glucagon and insulin, are responsible for breaking down the food that enters the stomach, turning it into fuel that can be used by the body, and then distributing it to the various parts of the body that need the fuel. The insulin-producing cells make up most of the islets. Glucagon works by increasing blood glucose levels while insulin works to decrease the blood glucose levels. Glucose that is in the blood is commonly called blood sugar. When

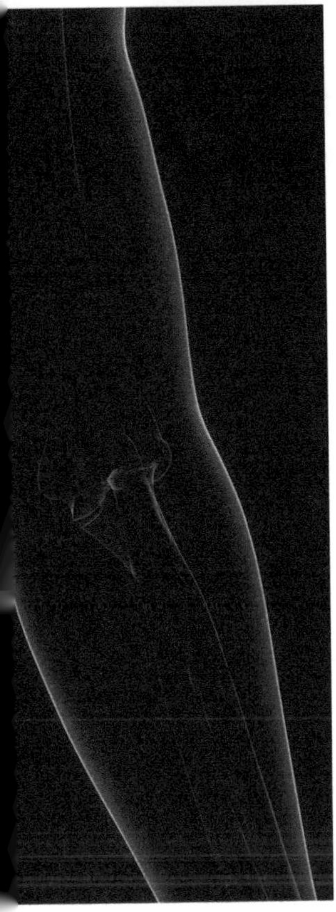

the alpha and beta cells work together properly, the body maintains a healthy amount of glucose, which is the main provider of energy for the majority of bodily functions. Most of the food people eat is converted into the simple sugar glucose. Glucose is not the same as the sugar found in food. When people talk about sugar in relation to diabetes, they really mean glucose. The glucose level in the blood fluctuates in response to a person's daily activities, from eating a meal to exercising to encountering stressful situations.

After a person eats a meal, the level of glucose in the body rises, and the body signals the pancreas to produce insulin. Insulin then signals muscle and fat tissue to absorb the amount of glucose needed for daily activities. Glucose that's not needed in the body at that time is stored in the liver in the form of a starch called glycogen. The body can access this reservoir of fuel whenever it's needed.

After a person exercises the body usually needs more fuel, so the alpha cells then become more active, producing glucagon. Glucagon breaks down the glycogen and causes it to be released into the bloodstream for the body to use. This raises the level of blood sugar. In healthy people, the level always falls into set values.

In a person without diabetes, the amount of insulin and glucagon produced is balanced. If, however, the glucose level increases and the body is unable to use the extra sugar because the level of insulin is insufficient or because the body can't absorb the insulin, then diabetes develops. Without enough insulin, cells can't use the glucose in the blood, and it builds up. The excess glucose can't be stored in the liver and muscles, and when the glucose in the blood reaches a certain level, the body will force it out as waste, increasing urination.

HISTORY OF DIABETES

Ancient Egyptians first described diabetes in writings dating to around 1500 BCE. In about 230 CE, a Greek physician named Aretaeus is believed to have called the disease "diabetes," which in Greek means "to siphon" or "to suck out." One of the symptoms of diabetes is excessive urination. He described diabetes as "the melting down of the flesh and limbs into urine." The word "diabetes" was used to describe how water seemed to pass right through the body of a person with the disease. Aretaeus wrote that a person with diabetes had an all-consuming thirst that resulted in constant urination. The urine of a person with diabetes contains a lot of extra sugar because the body is unable to break it down effectively. The word "mellitus," which is Latin for "honey," was added in 1679 to the term "diabetes" when a doctor tasted the urine of a person diagnosed with the disease and said it was as sweet as honey.

Although diabetes had been around a long time, it was not until the mid-1800s that medical science began to understand more accurately what it was and began to develop ways to treat it. Until the 20th century, if a person had diabetes, he or she usually died from it. Today, doctors know more about diabetes and how to help those with the condition live normal and healthy lives.

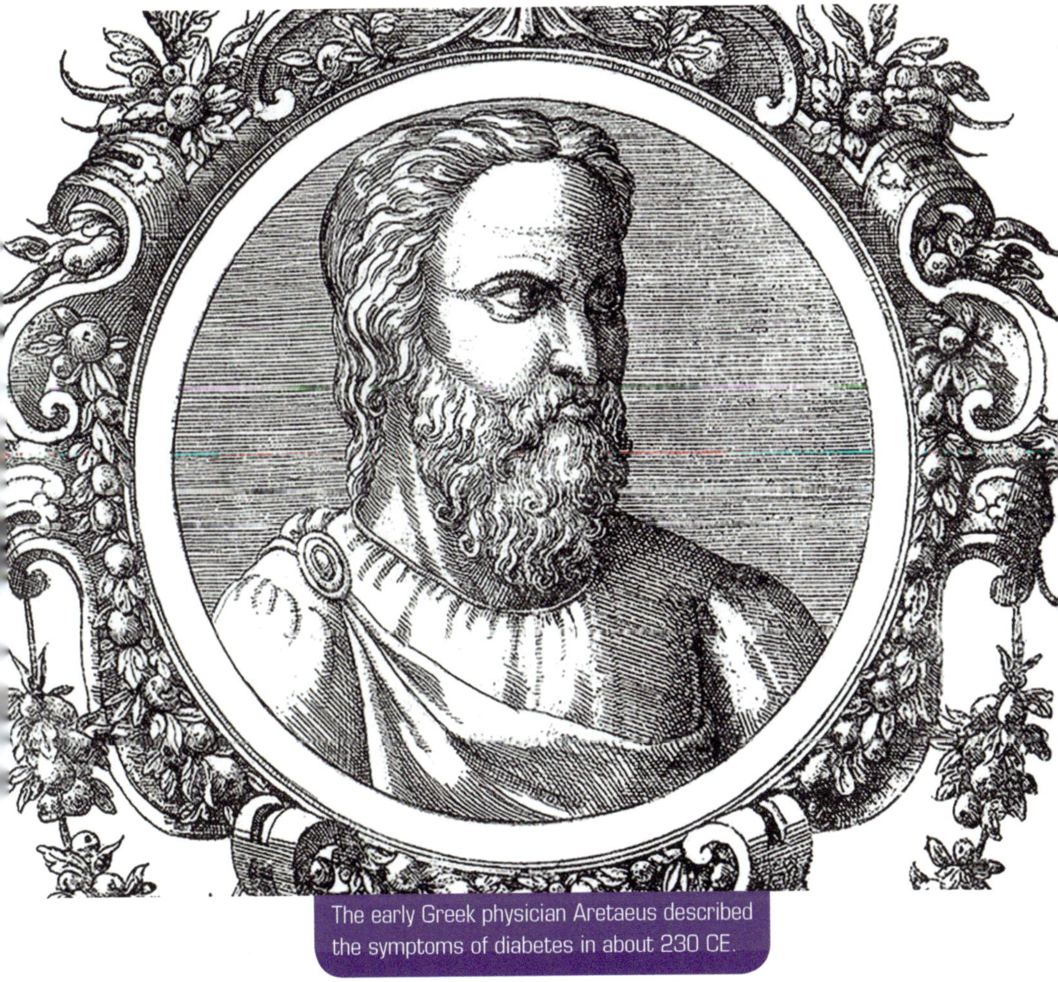

The early Greek physician Aretaeus described the symptoms of diabetes in about 230 CE.

TYPES OF DIABETES

There are two main types of diabetes. Type 1 depends on insulin for treatment and is called insulin-dependent diabetes. Type 2 is non-insulin dependent diabetes.

TYPE 1 DIABETES

Type 1 diabetes is an autoimmune disorder that can appear at any time in life. It stems from the destruction of the insulin-producing cells in the pancreas. The body produces little or no insulin and is unable to lower the level of glucose. Glucose accumulates in the blood, raising a person's blood sugar level. This is called hyperglycemia or high blood sugar. When the blood sugar level gets too high, glucose is removed from the body in urine as waste. As a result, someone with high blood sugar may have to go to the bathroom as often as his or her body needs to get rid of extra glucose. Frequent urination can result in a substantial loss of water, because water is a main component of urine. This water loss, known as dehydration, can lead to great thirst, dry mouth, blurry vision, and dry skin.

Also, if cells can't get the glucose they need, they "starve." This may make a diabetic person feel very hungry even when he or she has just finished eating. If someone has diabetes, his or her body doesn't produce the fuel it needs, and that person may often feel weak and tired. Weight loss also may occur as the body's demands for fuel force fat cells to break

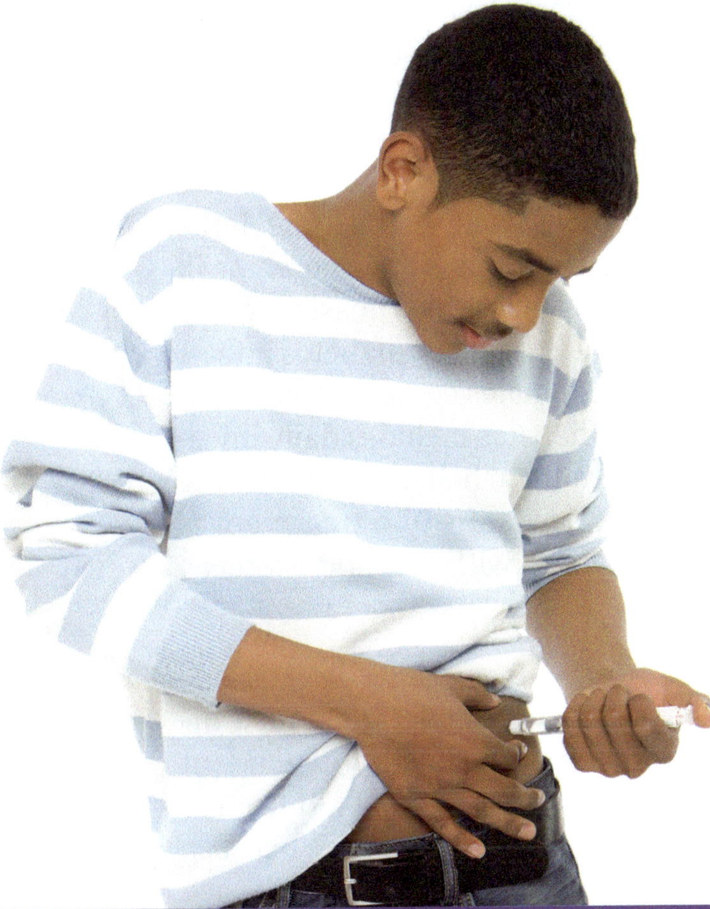

To treat his diabetes, this young man injects insulin from an insulin pen into his abdomen.

down. High glucose levels can damage nerves, which may result in a tingling feeling in the feet or leg cramps at night. It also interferes with the action of white blood cells, which can slow the healing of cuts. High glucose levels make it easier for bacteria to grow and may result in a variety of skin and urinary tract infections.

If hyperglycemia isn't treated, the result can be diabetic ketoacidosis (DKA) coma. When there's not enough insulin, the body looks for alternative fuel. That alternative fuel is fat. When fat is broken down into energy, it produces a poisonous waste called ketones. Ketones accumulate in the blood and eventually in the urine. If the condition isn't treated, the person will lose consciousness and possibly die.

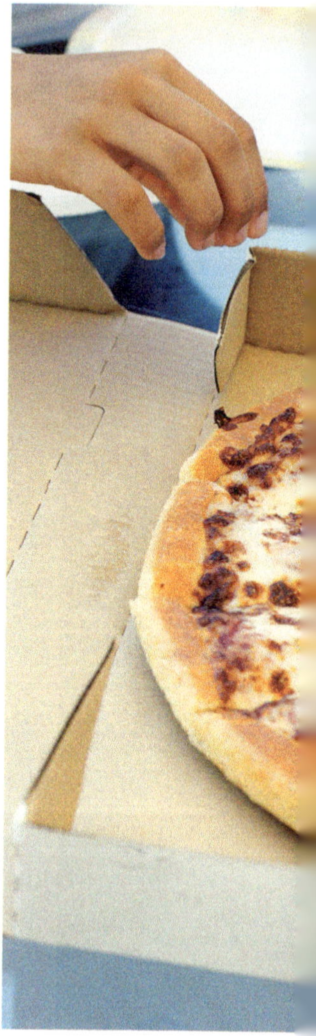

Insulin-dependent diabetes affects males and females equally. Treatment for type 1 diabetes includes daily injections of insulin to help the body use the glucose it needs. Insulin treatment is often balanced with diet and exercise.

TYPE 2 DIABETES

Type 2 diabetes also is called insulin-resistant or non–insulin-dependent diabetes mellitus (NIDDM). It used to be called adult-onset diabetes because it typically occurs in adults over the age of 40. As with type 1 diabetes, doctors realized that type 2 diabetes could appear at any age. Type 2 diabetes often, but not always, strikes those who are overweight or obese, or have a family history of the disease. In Type 2 diabetes, the body doesn't produce enough insulin, or it produces enough insulin but doesn't use it properly or resists it. Type 2 diabetes affects mostly females but can affect males as well.

Setting up a healthy diet and exercise plan for the patient is the usual treatment for this type of diabetes. For overweight people with type 2 diabe-

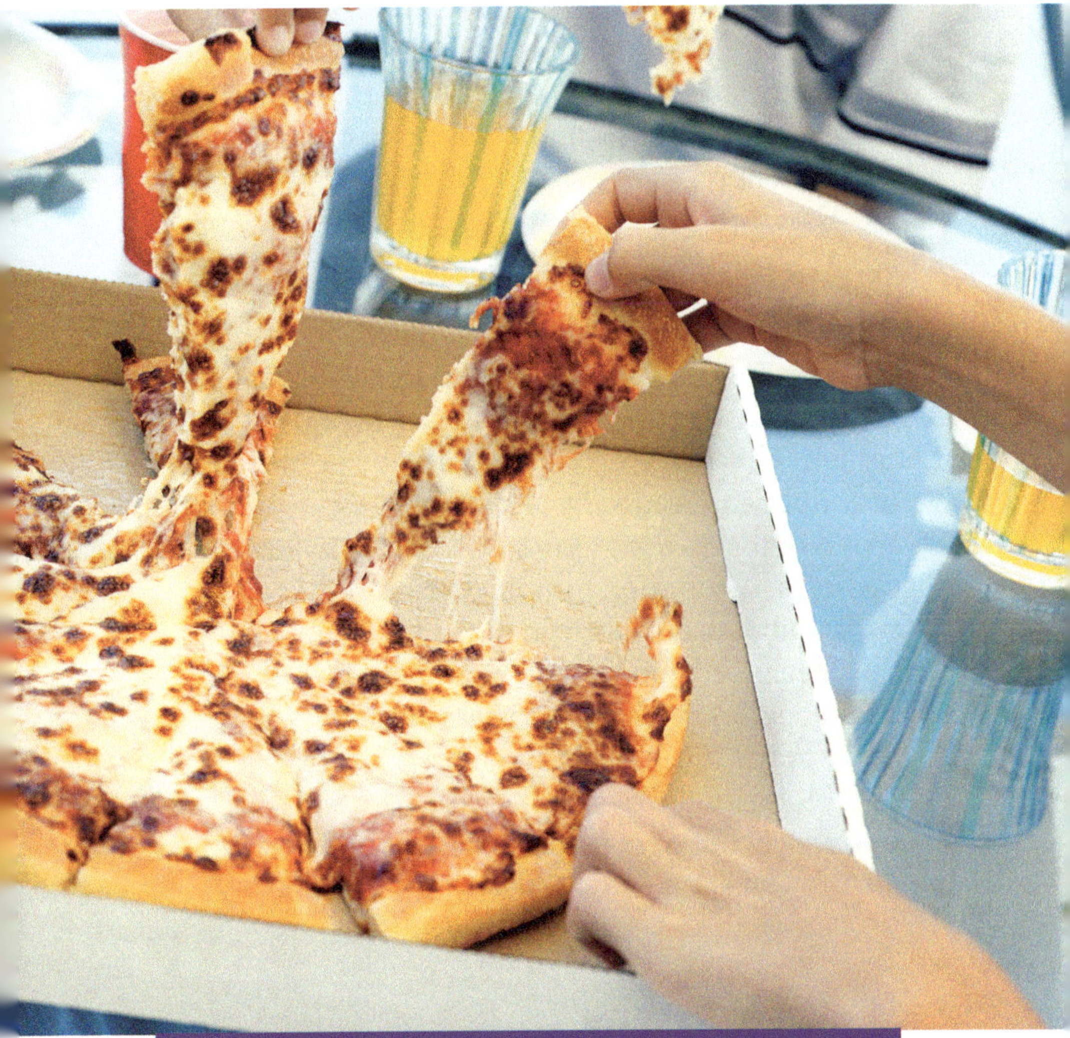

Fast food may be contributing to the rise in type 2 diabetes in young people.

tes, weight loss often helps the body use the insulin better. Some people with type 2 diabetes are also treated with insulin.

Millions of people have type 2 diabetes, and health care professionals are alarmed at the increasing number of young people who are developing this disease. In today's world, junk food, fast food, sodas, and foods high in calories seem to be part of the everyday diet of many young people, at home and in school.

BRITTLE DIABETES

Brittle diabetes, also called unstable diabetes or labile diabetes, occurs when a person's blood sugar level goes from one extreme to another for no apparent reason. This rising and falling can't be predicted and may not be preceded by any symptoms. People with type 1 diabetes are at greater risk for having brittle diabetes. A common misconception is that all teens with diabetes have brittle diabetes. People assume this because blood glucose levels often fluctuate during puberty. These fluctuations, however, aren't the same as those that characterize brittle diabetes. The blood sugar of people with brittle diabetes is frequently out of control.

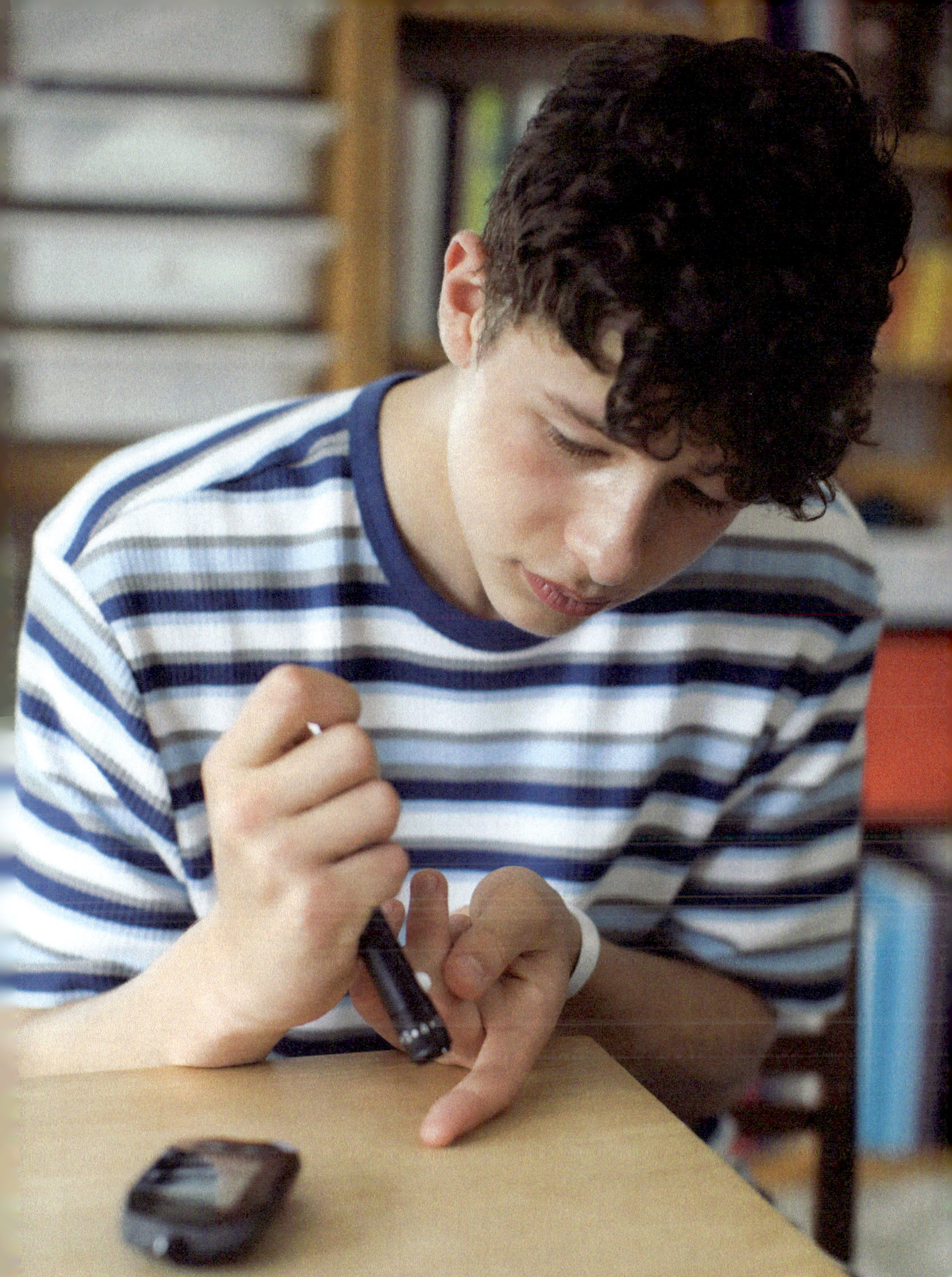

This young man prepares to stick his finger to test his blood sugar.

CHAPTER 2

DIAGNOSING DIABETES

Many people are unaware of the symptoms of diabetes. It's important to recognize these symptoms, especially if someone in your family has any type of diabetes or if you've had these symptoms for more than a short time. If you or someone you know experiences any of these symptoms, seek medical attention immediately. Many people who have diabetes, especially type 2 diabetes, are unaware they have the disease. If it's not treated properly, diabetes can be fatal. The sooner you find out, the sooner you can treat the condition.

TESTING FOR DIABETES

Not everyone who has diabetes has all, or even some, of these symptoms. The only way to be sure is to be tested for diabetes by a doctor. The general symptoms that many people with diabetes experience include:

- Frequent urination
- Continual thirst or dry mouth
- Always feeling hungry

- Tiredness and weakness
- Weight loss
- Blurry vision
- Numbness or tingling in feet or legs
- Skin infections or slow-to-heal cuts
- Extremely dry skin
- Irritability

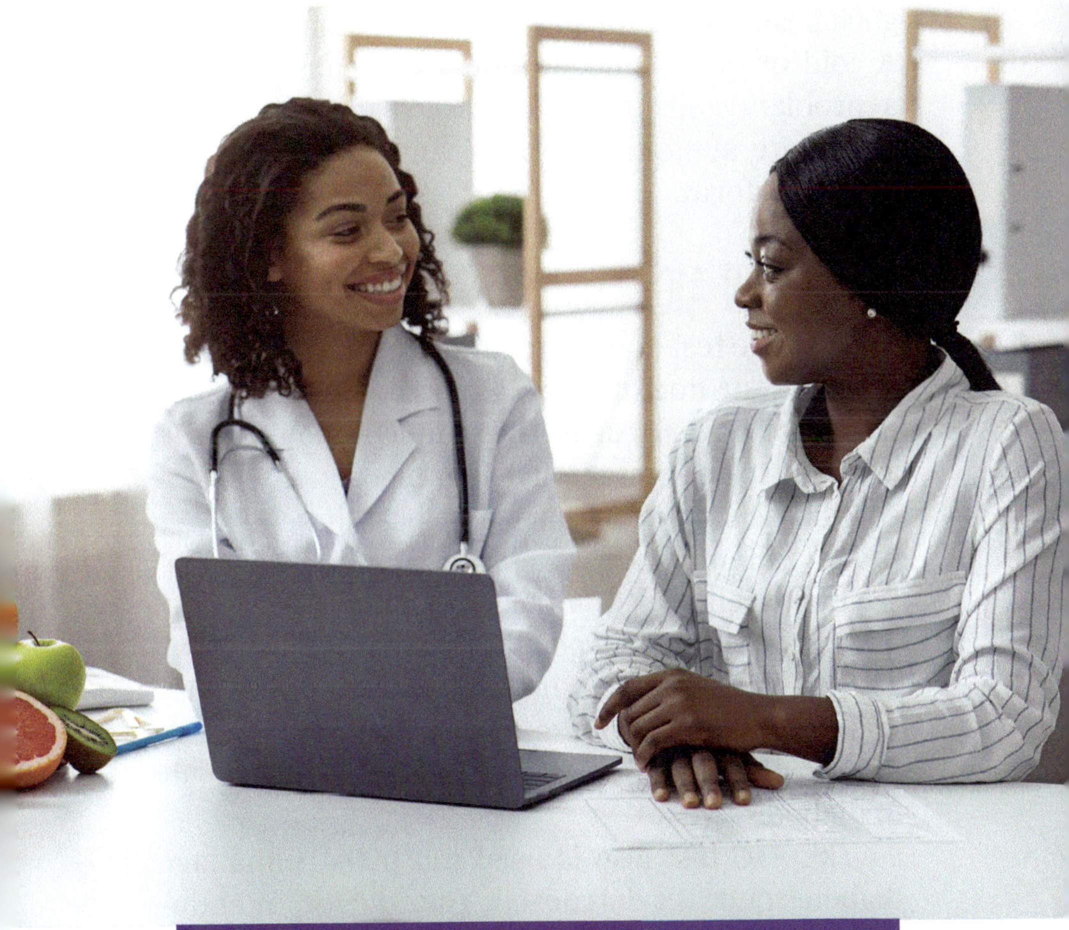

If you have any of the symptoms of diabetes, talk with your doctor about it. They can run tests and help you determine if you have diabetes or another condition and can help get you the treatment you need.

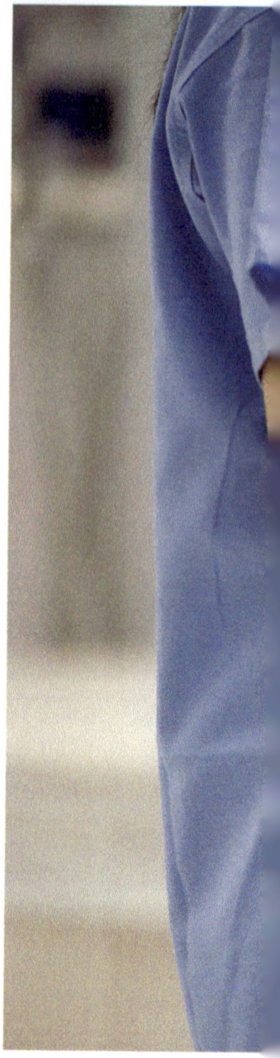

When you visit your doctor, you may be asked to have a screening test. A screening test requires a drop of blood and can tell your doctor if you might have diabetes. If this test indicates that diabetes is likely, the doctor will then perform a diagnostic test that will determine for certain whether you have diabetes. You should be in relatively good health when you have these tests done. A cold or other kind of illness can cause a problem getting the correct readings. These are some of the tests your doctor might perform.

HEMOGLOBIN A1C TEST (A1C)

This simple test doesn't require any preparation. Your doctor takes a blood sample from your finger or arm. The sample is then analyzed to determine what your blood glucose levels have been during the past three months. Hemoglobin is a protein found in red blood cells. Sugar attaches to hemoglobin at higher levels in people with diabetes. The percentage of red blood cells containing sugar-coated hemoglobin is measured with this test. A percentage of 6.5 or above indicates a diagnosis of diabetes.

The A1C test also is used routinely to manage diabetes once it's diagnosed. Your doctor, or endocrinologist, will order this test twice a year or as often as needed. The A1C number is your average

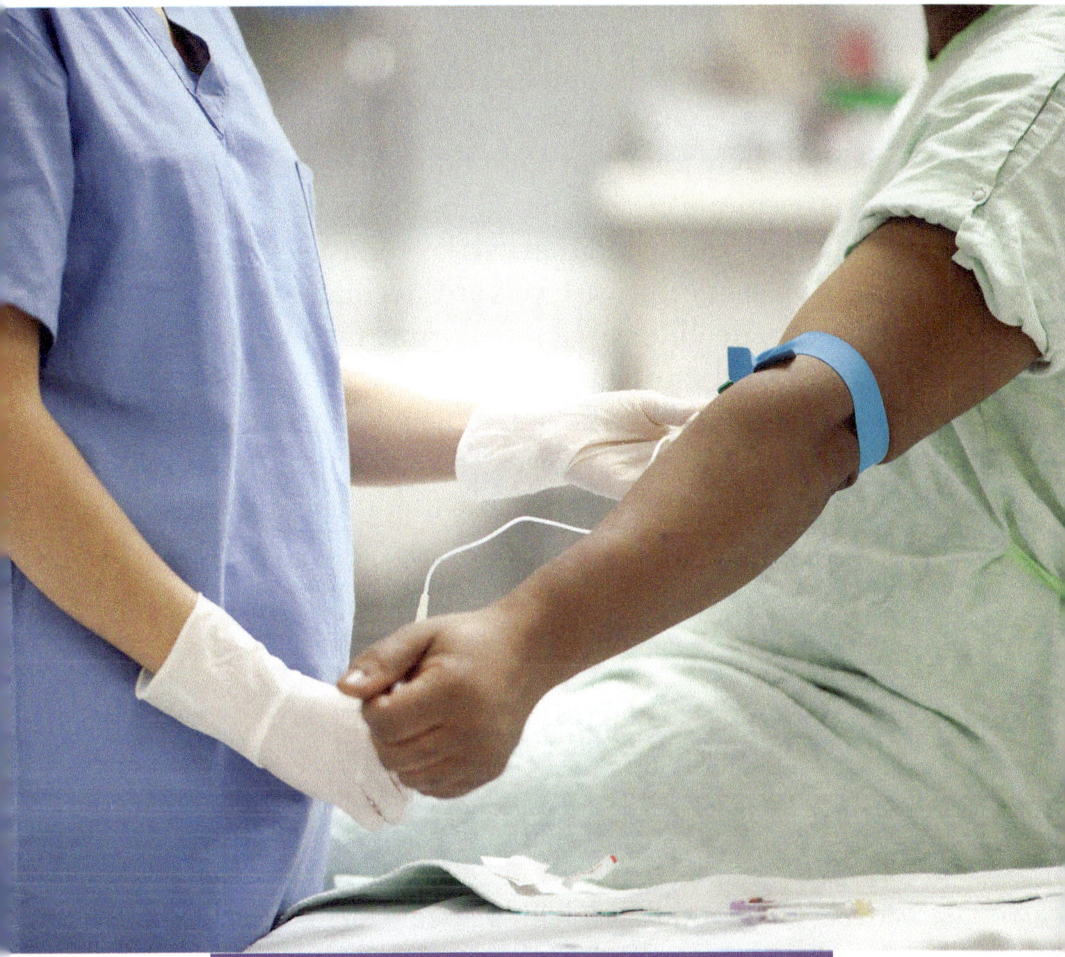

To diagnose diabetes, a sample of blood is taken to be analyzed.

glucose level similar to the numbers recorded on your glucose monitor. An A1C of 7 percent is a reading of about 154 milligrams of sugar per deciliter (mg/dl) on your meter. A deciliter is 1/10 of a liter. A milligram is 1/1000 of a gram. (A paper clip weighs a gram.) A1C numbers higher than 6.5 are linked to diabetes complications.

FASTING PLASMA GLUCOSE TEST (FPG)

For this test, you don't eat or drink anything overnight, usually for about eight hours. Then the doctor takes a sample of your blood for analysis. Plasma is the part of your blood that carries solid cells. Normal fasting plasma glucose levels are less than 100 mg/dl. For every deciliter of blood, normal fasting glucose levels should show less than 99 milligrams. If the test is higher than that, the doctor will do the test again.

With the new American Diabetes Association guidelines, doctors believe fasting plasma glucose levels above 126 mg/dl indicates the possibility of diabetes.

ORAL GLUCOSE TOLERANCE TEST (OGTT)

Some doctors may recommend an oral glucose tolerance test. You must fast overnight before this test as well. The doctor will check your blood glucose level. Then you'll be given a sugary drink and your blood glucose level will be checked again in one hour, then again two hours after the first test, and then again three hours after the second test. A person without diabetes will show a quick rise and fall in glucose levels after the drink. This is a result of the infusion of glucose and then the insulin response. A person with diabetes will show a rise that doesn't come down very quickly, indicating insufficient or lack of insulin or impaired glucose tolerance. If your doctor suspects diabetes, additional tests might be ordered to make a diagnosis.

WHO GETS DIABETES?

Although some people are more likely to get diabetes than others, diabetes can affect anyone at any time. About 34.2 million people in the United States, or 10 percent of the population, have diabetes. Five percent of the population has no idea they have the disease. Consider these interesting statistics:

- Each year, 1.5 million new cases of diabetes in people ages 18 or older are diagnosed.
- Between 5 and 10 percent of all cases of diabetes are type 1.
- About 90 to 95 percent of all cases of diabetes are type 2.
- Nine out of ten diabetic Americans have type 2 diabetes.

Type 1 diabetes is most often found in young people. It's called insulin-dependent diabetes because people need to give themselves insulin shots to stay healthy. Sometimes it's called juvenile diabetes or juvenile-onset diabetes because it usually starts in childhood. It's not known how to prevent type 1 diabetes, although scientists are researching this.

Type 2 diabetes is on the rise and usually appears in people who are 40 years old or older, have a family history of diabetes, are overweight and do not exercise regularly, had gestational diabetes, or are of certain racial and ethnic groups (most commonly African American, Hispanic American, Asian and Pacific Islander, and Native American). Many cases of type 2 diabetes can be prevented and possibly reversed by following a strict diet and exercising.

Diabetes also can be caused by factors such as another chronic illness, genetic syndromes, malnutrition, drugs, and surgery.

DISCOVERY OF INSULIN

In 1910, Dr. Edward Sharpey-Schafer of Scotland decided that a chemical he called insulin was missing from the pancreas of people with diabetes. In 1921, at the University of Toronto, doctors Frederick Banting and Charles Best believed that insulin was manufactured in the pancreas in cells called the islets of Langerhans. To investigate this idea, they first removed the pancreas from healthy dogs, causing them to develop diabetes. Then they took fluid from the islets of Langerhans in healthy dogs—those that still had their pancreas—and injected it into the sick dogs. The effect on the sick dogs was dramatic: It stopped their symptoms.

Banting and Best then teamed up with J. B. Collip to extract a more refined form of insulin from cattle. Under the direction of Dr. J.J.R. Macleod, these four men developed insulin as a treatment for diabetes. That same year, an oral dose of insulin was tested on

Dr. Joe Gilchrist. Nothing seemed to happen. Early the next year, Leonard Thompson, a patient at Toronto Hospital, was injected with insulin on two different occasions and his condition improved. In May of 1922, Macleod officially announced the discovery of insulin.

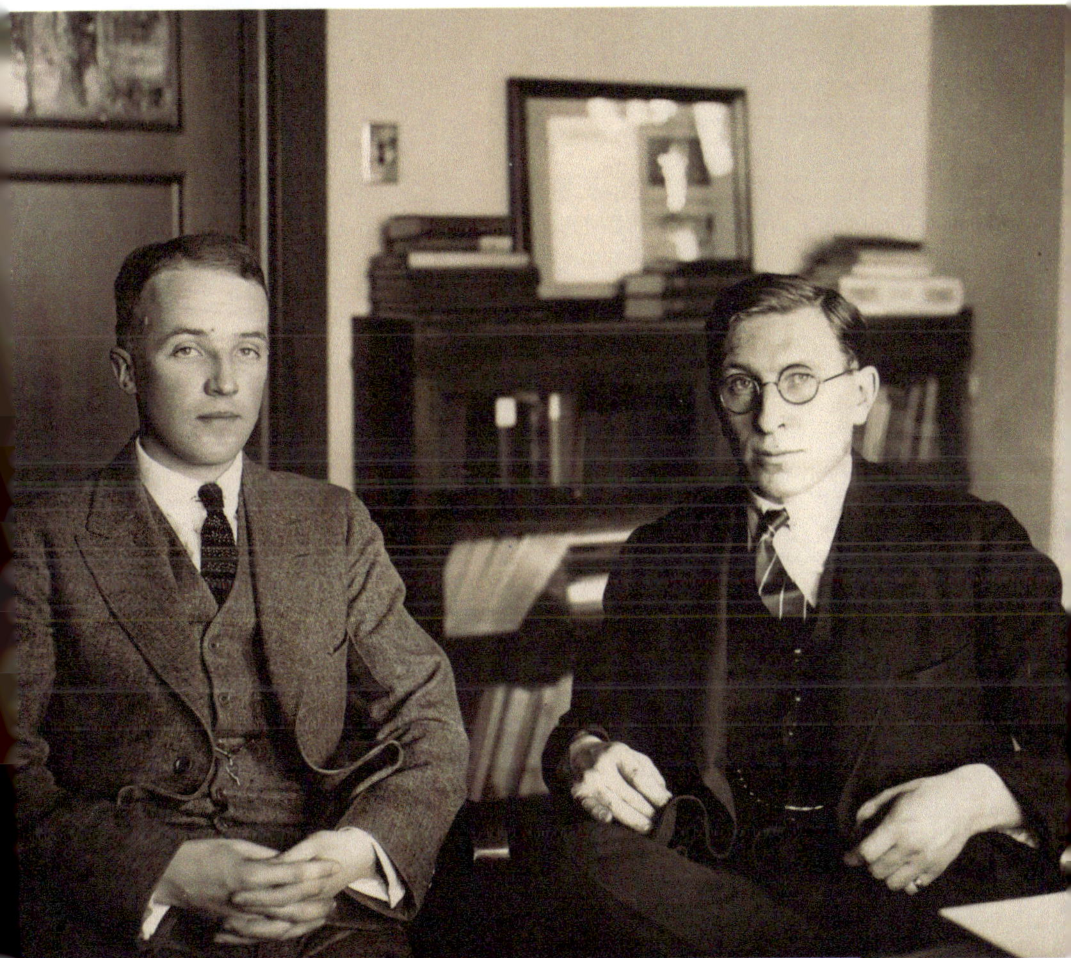

Doctors Charles Best and Frederick Banting, shown here in 1924, discovered that insulin is manufactured in the pancreas.

DIABETES AND GENETICS

Having someone with diabetes in your family increases your chances of developing diabetes. If you have a sibling or a parent with type 1 diabetes, your chance of developing it is about 10 to 25 percent

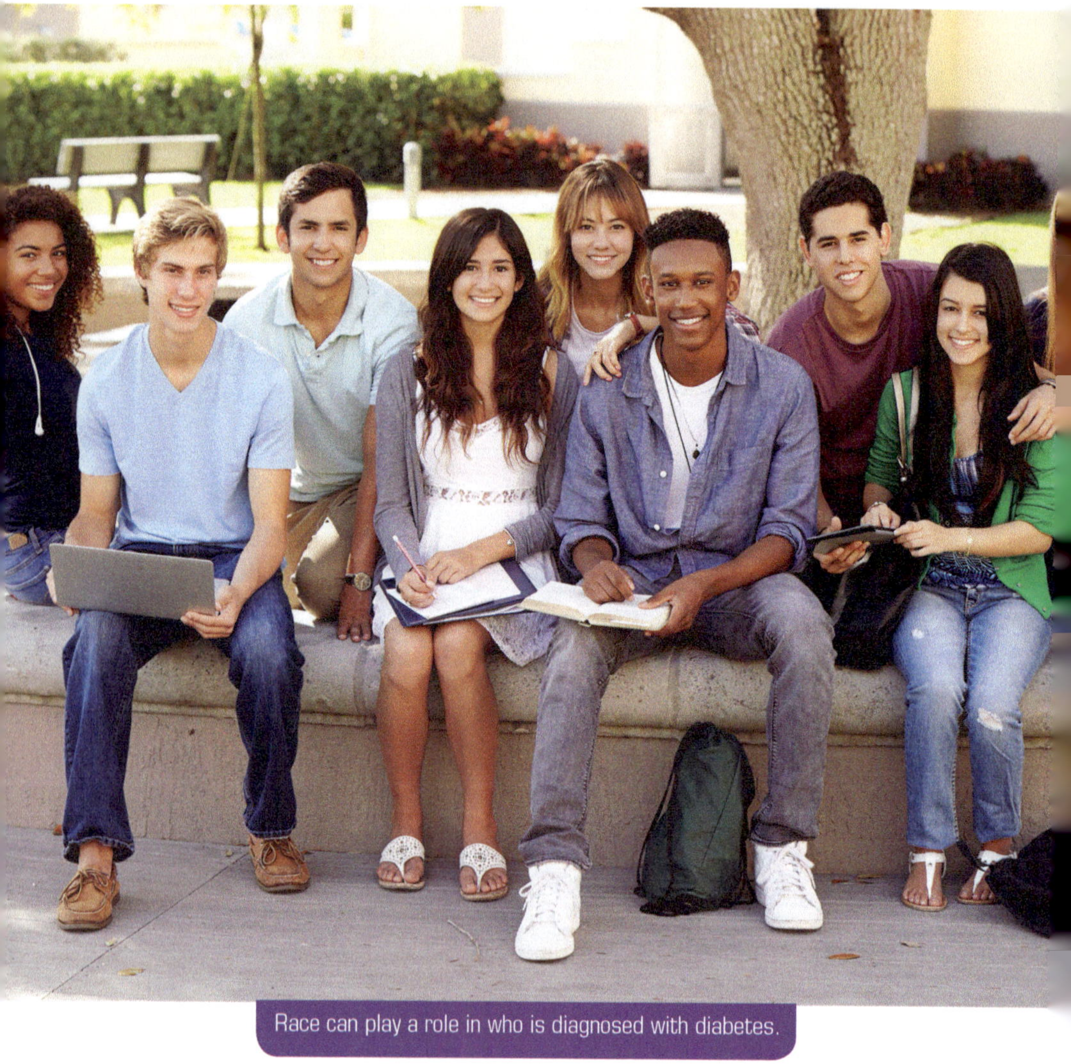

Race can play a role in who is diagnosed with diabetes.

higher than the average person because you may have inherited a family tendency toward diabetes. If your identical twin has diabetes, your chance of developing it increases to between 25 and 50 percent more than the average person. Researchers are looking into how environmental triggers might result in a diagnosis in people with a genetic predisposition to type 1 and type 2 diabetes.

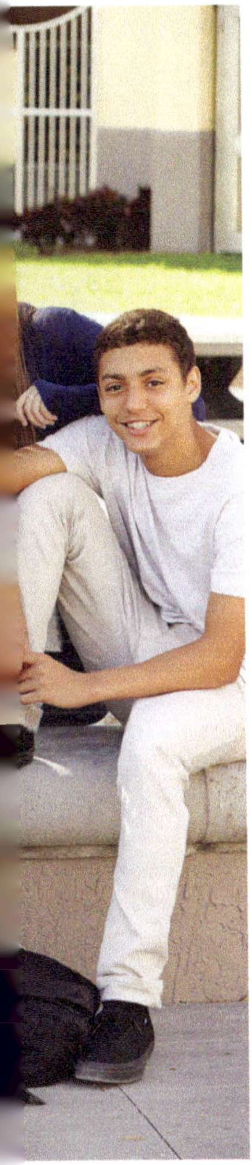

DIABETES AND RACE

People all over the world are diagnosed with diabetes every day and race can play a role. Here's a sampling of Americans diagnosed with diabetes:

- Non-Hispanic whites: 7.5 percent
- Asian Americans: 9.2 percent
- African Americans: 11.7 percent
- Hispanic Americans: 12.5 percent
- Native Americans: 14.7 percent

FEELINGS ABOUT DIABETES

When you're first diagnosed with diabetes, you might experience a range of emotions: denial, anger, guilt, depression, grief, and fear. These feelings are normal, can come in any order, and return from time to time. They become a problem only when they're not followed by acceptance and the desire to move forward and cope with diabetes. That way you can live a long and productive life, as do many people with diabetes.

Managing your diabetes can seem like a tiresome chore. But the more you learn about the disease and how to manage it well, the easier it will become. Currently, diabetes can't be cured, but monitoring your blood glucose, eating a healthy diet, and exercising can help you prevent the risk of complications and early death. You're in control of your diabetes and your future with it.

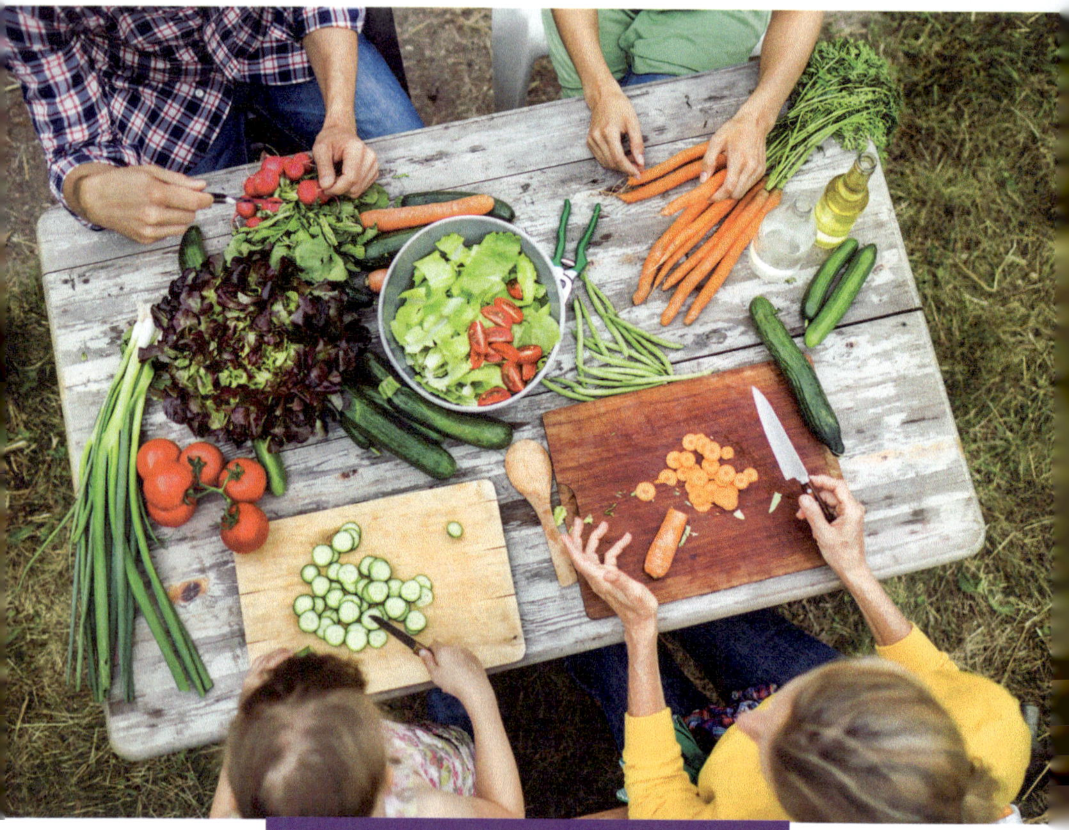

Eating a healthy diet is important for people with diabetes and can help avoid long-term complications.

10 GREAT QUESTIONS TO ASK AFTER YOU HAVE BEEN DIAGNOSED WITH DIABETES

1. Which doctors or specialists should I see to stay healthy with diabetes?
2. Which foods will affect my blood glucose levels?
3. How will I know when my blood glucose level is too high or too low?
4. What supplies should I carry and whom should I call in an emergency?
5. Does insulin and other diabetes medication have side effects?
6. How do I manage my blood glucose levels when I'm sick?
7. How can I avoid long-term complications of diabetes?
8. Should I tell my friends and classmates that I have diabetes?
9. Can I still do activities such as sports or driving a car?
10. Will diabetes prevent me from having children and will they inherit the disease?

CHAPTER 3

ADJUSTING TO LIFE WITH DIABETES

Having diabetes requires you to adjust your daily routine to successfully treat it. You need to schedule time to monitor your blood sugar, use insulin as needed for the food you eat, test your urine for ketones, and keep a daily log of these results. You also will need to pay more attention to your diet and exercise or sports. Doctor visits also will have to be worked into your schedule. You will have to accept more responsibility for your health by working with your health care team and learning more about the disease.

ISSUES THAT AFFECT DIABETES

Several issues that affect diabetics make it hard to accept the daily changes to life. There's daily testing and insulin usage, perhaps feeling different, watching diet and getting exercise, and worrying about getting sick or even dying.

Daily testing and administering insulin by a pump or pen injection might be uncomfortable, but these processes take only a few minutes out of your day. If the injection site hurts, try rubbing it with an ice cube. Also, it helps to pinch a section of the site when you inject the pen or syringe. If one site hurts, try another and rotate the injection sites you use.

If you're afraid that having diabetes makes you different somehow, remember that more than 34 million Americans have diabetes. If someone makes hurtful assumptions or comments because

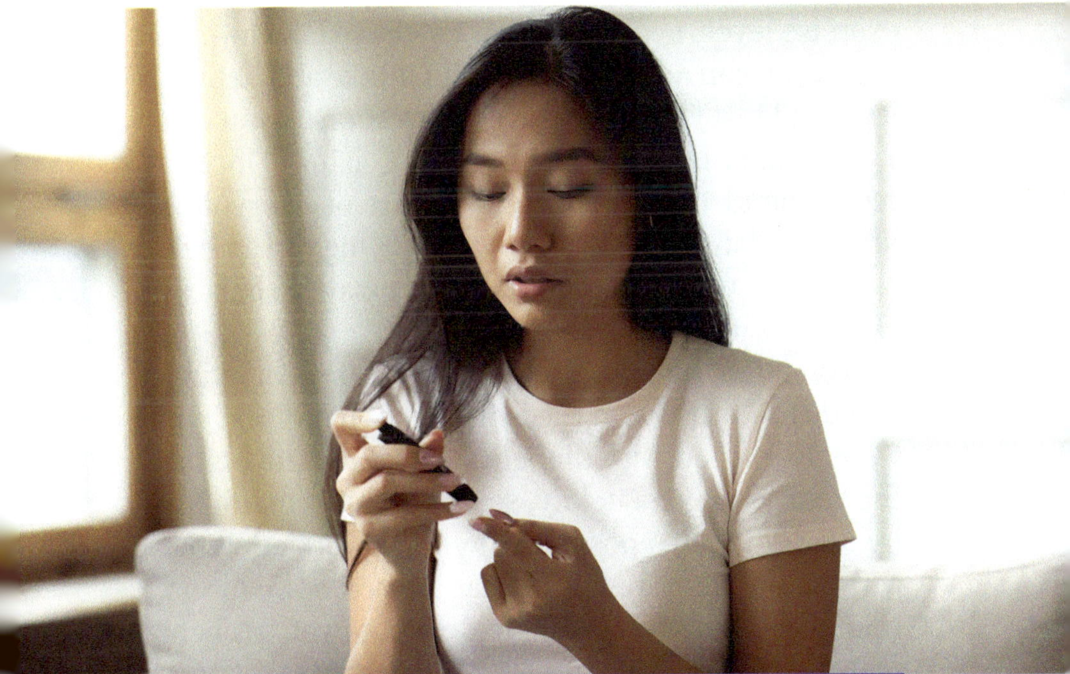

At first, it might seem scary to have to stick yourself with a needle to test your blood sugar or inject insulin, but you will get used to doing it. There are also ways to manage any pain you might feel from the needle sticks.

you have diabetes, it shows that he or she lacks knowledge about the disease.

You might be concerned about what to eat or that you might eat the wrong foods. A healthy diet includes everything you've already been eating, but in moderation. You can still have a piece of pie now and then, but you have to balance your insulin intake with it. Your health care team might include a dietitian who can help you plan healthy and delicious meals. If you have type 2 diabetes, diet and exercise are the main methods for controlling blood sugar.

You might be worried about going out to eat or eating at someone's house. If you know your schedule ahead of time, you can plan your insulin intake and exercise levels accordingly. If you have last-minute plans, you can adjust your insulin intake and activity level and test your glucose levels as soon as you can.

You may be worried about exercising. Doctors recommend that exercise be a part of everyone's life, not just people with diabetes. One of the best exercises is walking. As with diet, you have to balance exercise with insulin intake.

You might be worried about getting sick or dying. Before the 1920s and the isolation of insulin, if you were diagnosed with diabetes you would die before the year was out. Luckily, scientists have made living with diabetes possible. If you're worried about getting sick as a result of diabetes complications, remember that you can help delay or even prevent many of the complications by taking control of your diabetes now.

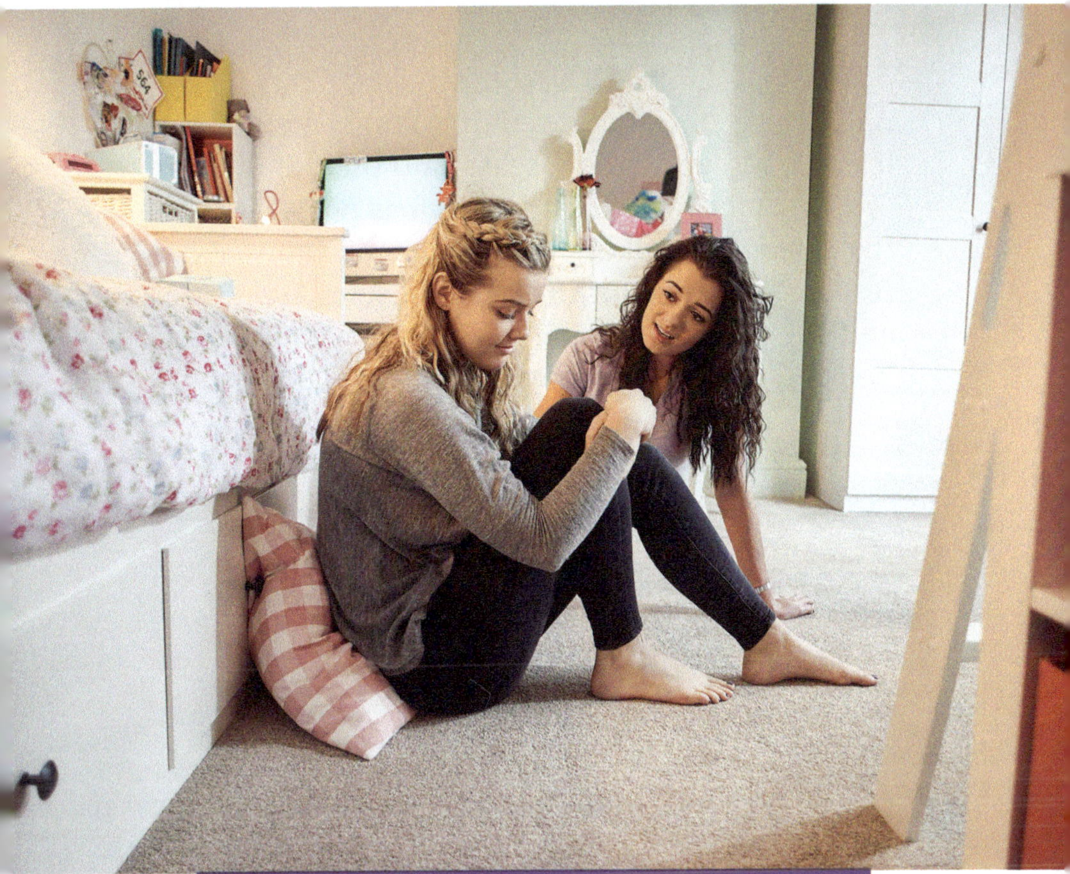

While it might be normal for a person with diabetes to worry about their condition, too much worry and stress can raise blood glucose.

Although it's normal to worry about having diabetes, too much worry can cause unnecessary stress. Too much stress from worry, anxiety, depression, anger, guilt, or even a physical ailment can increase blood sugar levels and lead to hyperglycemia. Just as you can take control of your diabetes, you can take control of your stress. People with diabetes live long, full, and productive lives if they take care of themselves.

HOW DIABETES AFFECTS YOUR FAMILY

A diagnosis of diabetes requires family members to learn to integrate the disease into their daily lives. The first step is to learn as much as possible about the disease by talking to your doctor and through resources such as the American Diabetes Association and the Juvenile Diabetes Research Foundation. You and your family members might want to join a

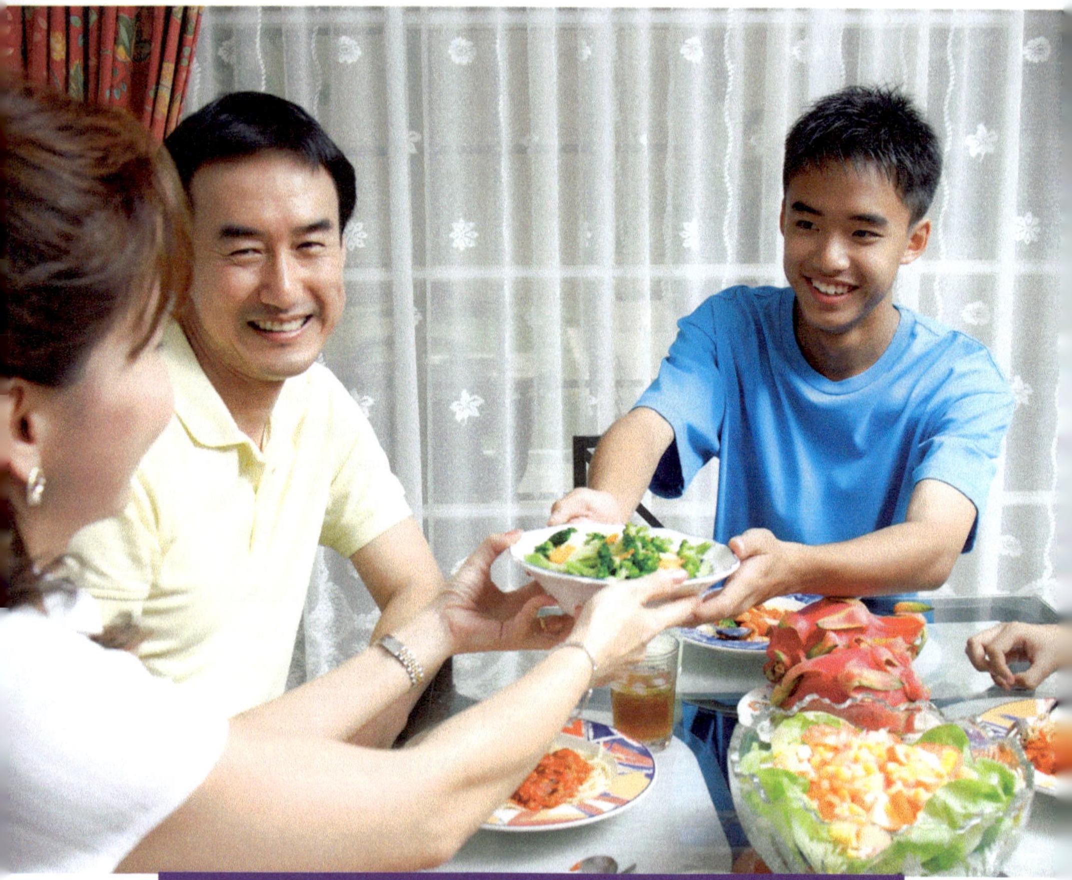

A healthy diet is good for the whole family, not just the person with diabetes.

CREATING A 504 PLAN

A 504 Plan is a document that helps to protect students with any disability from discrimination and ensures them the same rights to an education as any other student. It also provides for accommodations for students to manage their disability at school as needed. The 504 Plan is available to all students attending public and private schools.

Students with diabetes and their parents can set up a 504 Plan at school with their doctor's assistance. Each student and their 504 Plan is evaluated on an individual basis so that their specific needs can be met at school. Administrators, teachers, and the school nurse will learn how to help a student manage their disability in all school activities, and in the event of a school or personal emergency.

A 504 Plan offers students with diabetes a safe environment to check their blood glucose and administer insulin. The plan also accommodates students' doctor visits, sick days, and the right to make up schoolwork without penalty. A sample 504 Plan can be downloaded from the Internet.

diabetes support group to learn how other people in similar situations have handled the adjustment.

If your diabetes requires insulin injections, you and your parents have to learn how to do this. Everyone in the family should learn to recognize the warning signs of hypoglycemia and hyperglycemia and should know what to do in an emergency, including using a glucagon kit.

The family diet might be changed to accommodate diabetes, probably making it healthier for everyone.

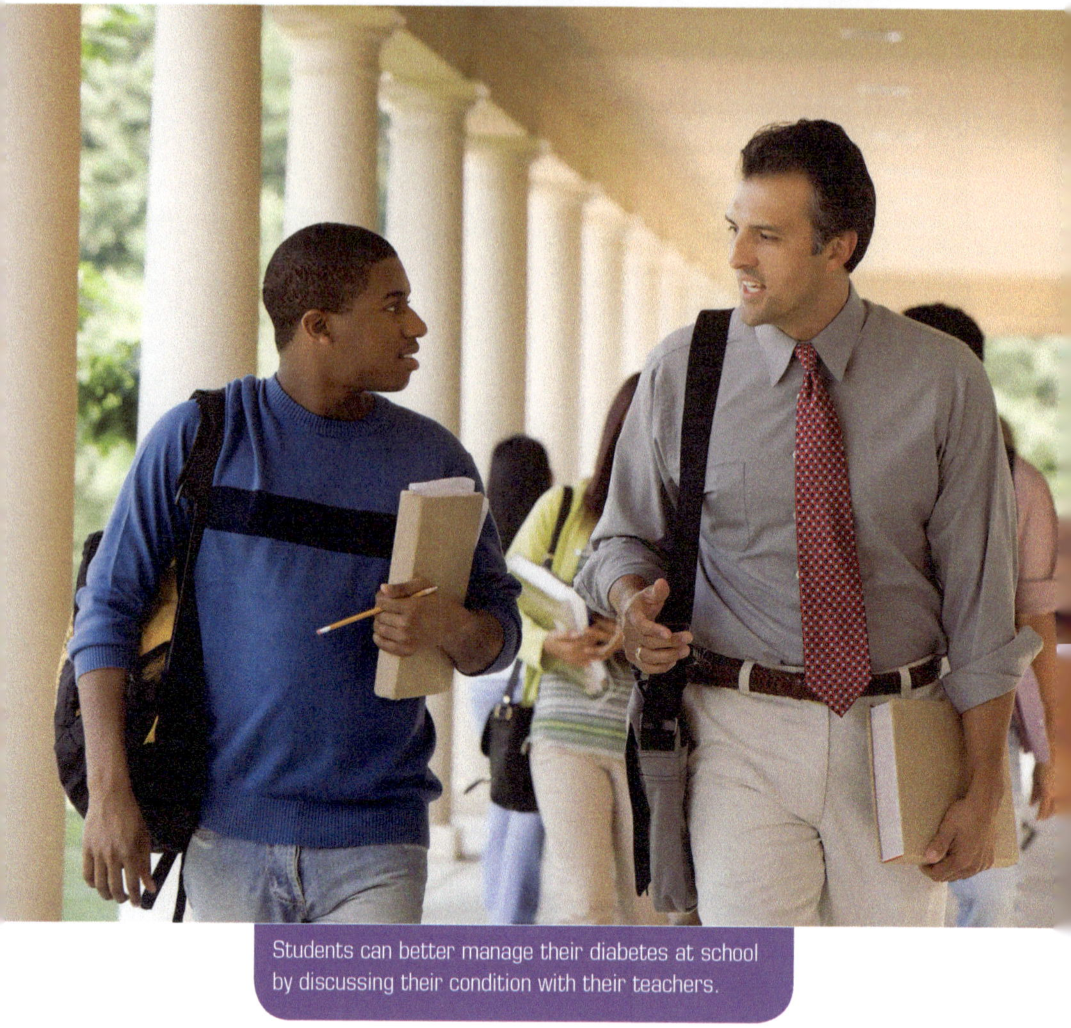

Students can better manage their diabetes at school by discussing their condition with their teachers.

HOW DIABETES AFFECTS YOUR EDUCATION

Your teachers and the school nurse need to know about your diabetes and your experience with it. This way, your teachers will understand when you need to test your blood sugar or give yourself an injection or if you need to eat a snack during class

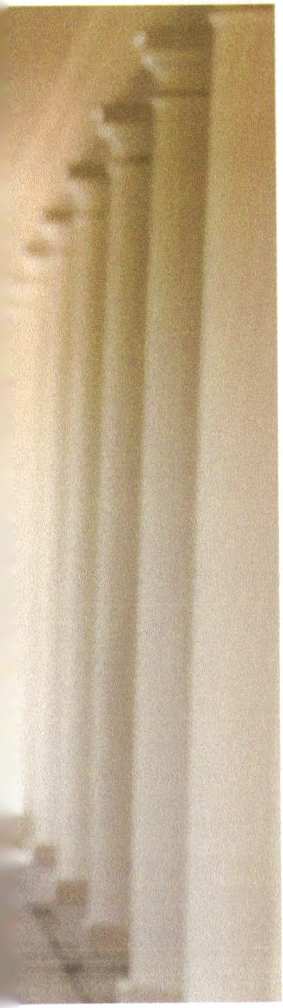

or in the nurse's office. You might want to research insulin pumps to see if pumping might be a good option for you. You also need to inform your teachers of the signs of hypoglycemia or hyperglycemia so they can help you if either of those conditions arise.

If you're involved in sports, you should tell your coach or physical education teacher. Because exercise affects glucose levels, they need to recognize the difference between hypoglycemia and hyperglycemia so that they can react to them in time.

Your classmates may ask you questions about diabetes and be curious about how you test your blood sugar and inject insulin. Eventually, it will seem as routine to them as it is to you. Explain to your friends that one of the signs of hypoglycemia is irritability so they may alert you to test your blood sugar. It's important to have a support network of teachers, friends, and family. Also, stand up for yourself if you're being treated unfairly or if hurtful things are being said about you.

Schools have a 504 Plan that protects students who have "a disability in one of life's functions." In the case of diabetes, the disability is the wide fluctuation in blood sugar. The 504 Plan also allows students to request accommodations due to missed days. This means your school is required to allow you to make up work missed without penalty.

MYTHS AND FACTS ABOUT DIABETES

- **MYTH #1**: Diabetes is caused by eating too much sugar.

- **FACT #1**: Diabetes is the result when your body doesn't make any or very little insulin and can't process the food you eat. Type 1 diabetes is an autoimmune disease and also can be inherited. Type 2 diabetes can result from an unhealthy lifestyle that includes obesity and lack of exercise.

- **MYTH #2**: People who have diabetes need to follow a special diet and can't eat certain foods.

- **FACT #2**: A healthy and balanced diet is good for everyone and is key in managing diabetes. You don't have to give up your favorite foods, but you should practice portion control, limit your indulgences, and take medication or insulin as prescribed for the food you eat.

- **MYTH #3**: If I use a continuous glucose meter and an insulin pump, the machines will manage my diabetes for me.

- **FACT #3:** Using newer technology, such as a continuous glucose meter and an insulin pump, makes it easier to manage diabetes. But it doesn't take the place of knowing what your blood glucose levels are, determining what you should and should not eat, and recognizing how much insulin your pump is administering.

- **MYTH #4:** If I have type 2 diabetes, I don't have to worry about avoiding sugar and fatty foods as long as I take my medication.

- **FACT #4:** Type 2 diabetes sometimes develops in people who are overweight and not active. Eating a healthy and balanced diet, exercising, and losing weight can help avoid complications such as cardiovascular disease and heart disease.

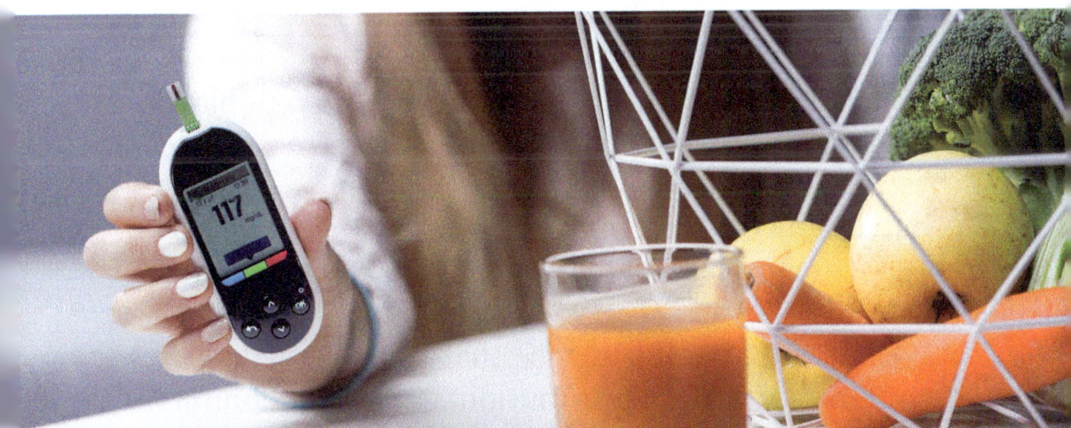

Newer technology makes it easier than ever to manage diabetes, but you still need to pay attention to your blood glucose levels. This can help you figure out if you should or should not eat something at that time.

CHAPTER 4

DIABETIC SUPPLIES AND TESTING

To monitor and control your diabetes, you need specific equipment. There are several different kinds and brands of equipment. Your doctor or diabetes educator can help you learn how they work, how to maintain them, and which ones your health insurance will cover.

GLUCOSE MONITORS

Standard glucose monitors tell you what your blood sugar is at the moment you take it. They're compact and can be carried in your pocket or purse. Continuous glucose monitors (CGM) measure your blood glucose throughout the day and night. They're small and can be carried on your body. Data can be downloaded to a mobile device that can then help you manage your diabetes. Continuous glucose monitors are especially helpful for people who have trouble keeping their blood sugar in range or can't sense a hypoglycemic episode.

Your doctor or health care team will determine the best glucose monitor for you. Check if your glucose monitor needs to be calibrated. This will ensure that your readings are correct. Always use fresh strips and supplies and keep your meter clean. Also, keep your meter away from extreme cold or hot temperatures.

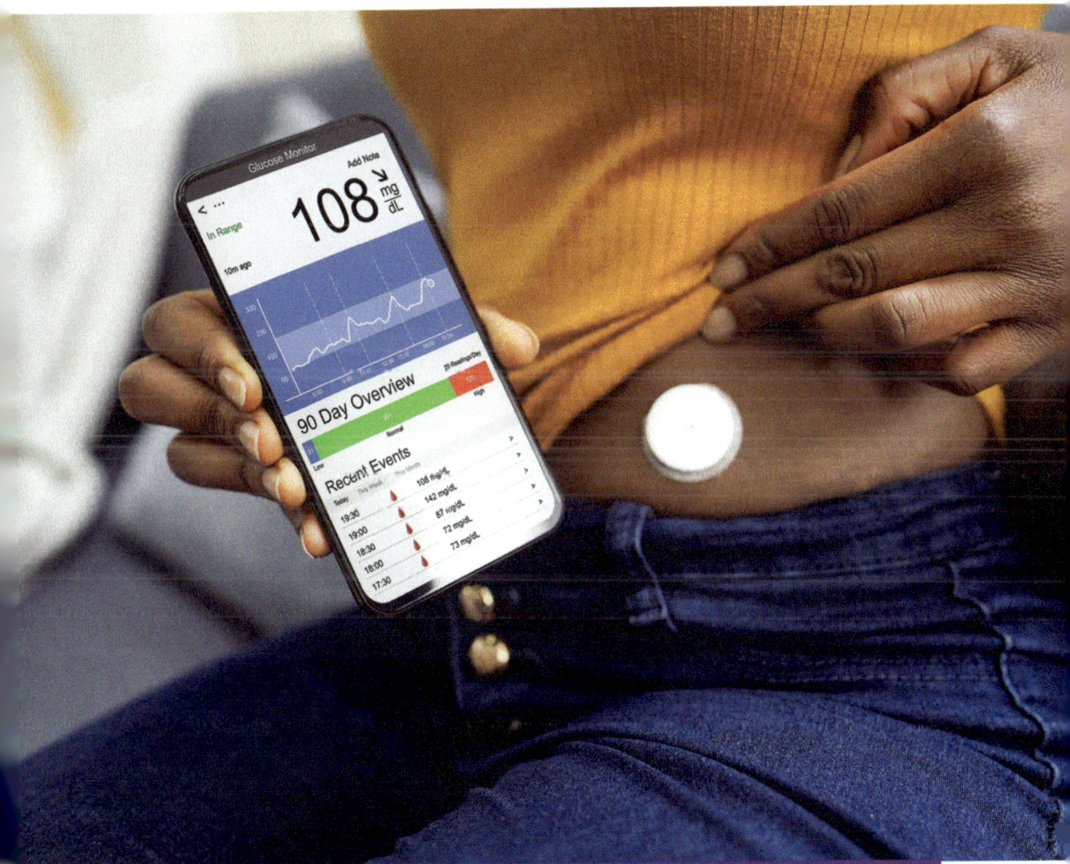

If you have a continuous glucose monitor, you may be able to download a special app on your phone that receives and displays the information collected by the monitor. This can make it easier to understand your diabetes.

INSULIN PENS

Insulin can be injected using a pen. Some pens use cartridges, like an ink pen, and some pens can be disposed of after the insulin is used up. The pen is easy to carry and easy to use. When you're ready to give yourself an injection, you wipe the top with alcohol, screw the needle onto the special end of the pen, prime the pen (that is, test it), set the correct dose, and then give yourself the injection.

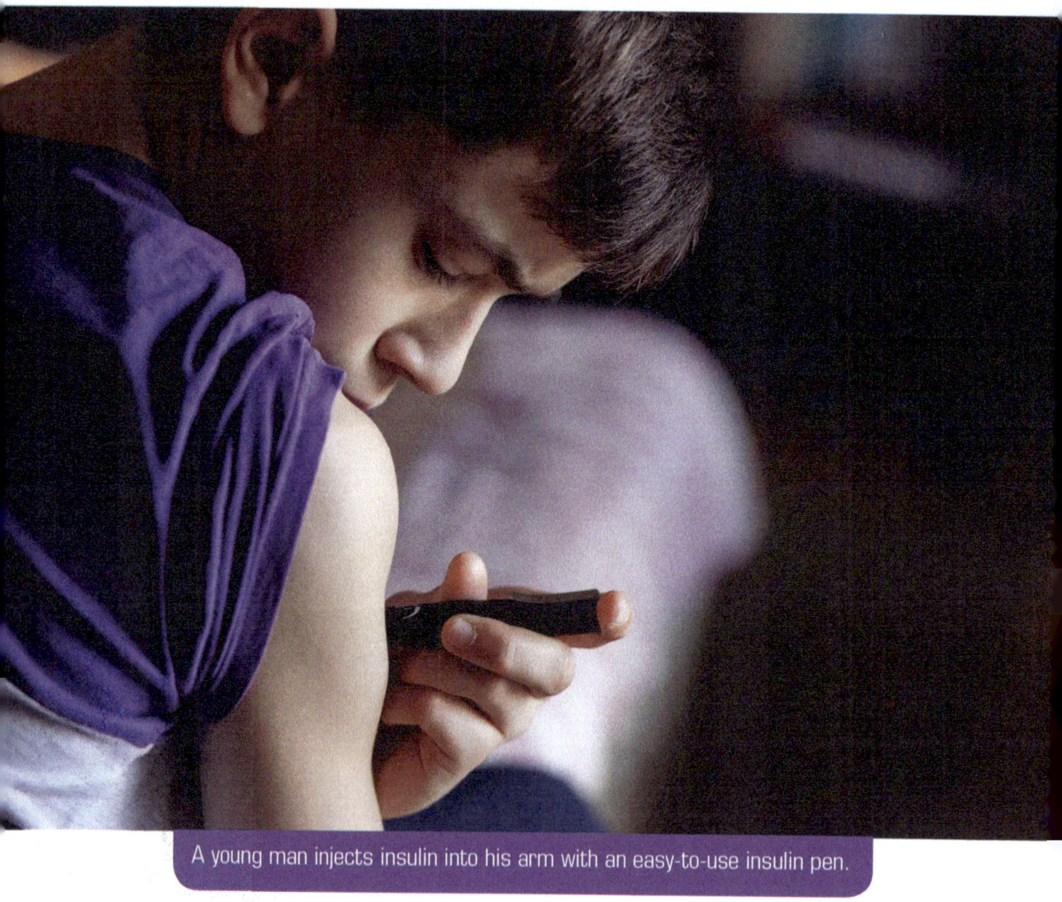

A young man injects insulin into his arm with an easy-to-use insulin pen.

PUMPS

Pumps are commonly used in type 1 diabetes to deliver insulin. A pump can increase your freedom because, when used properly, it provides better control over your diabetes. The pump reservoir holds the insulin, and the computer chip is programmed to deliver a certain amount of insulin.

The needle is placed under the skin, usually on the abdomen, where clothing won't interfere with it. You wear the pump even when you sleep. The pump administers small doses of insulin (basal dose) all day. This continuous delivery of insulin keeps blood glucose levels within normal ranges throughout the day and night. The pump is programmed to give larger doses of insulin (bolus dose) to balance out the food eaten. Because you control the insulin amount by simple programming, you can deliver different amounts of insulin without many injections. With a pump, you have only one injection when you change the infusion set.

Another way of administering insulin and measuring blood glucose is by a closed-loop system. This system pairs an insulin pump and a continuous glucose meter that communicate with each other. The pump then automatically adjusts the amount of insulin delivered

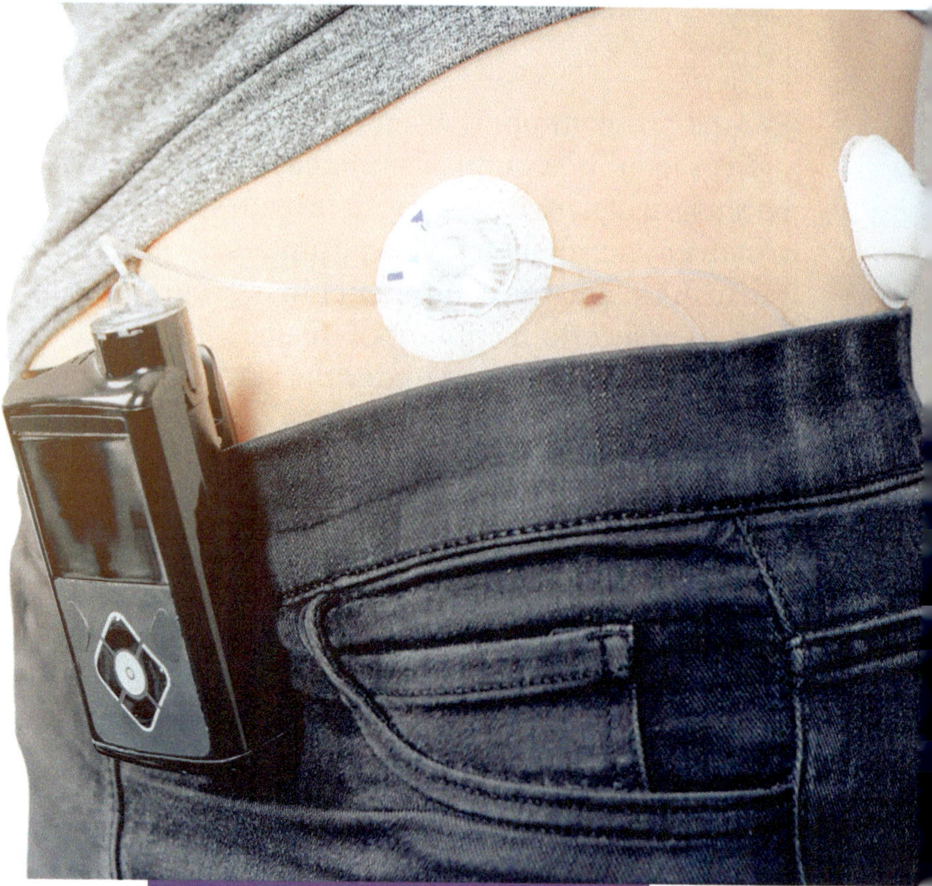

A person with diabetes can wear an infusion pump that's connected on the belly to deliver insulin.

based on the blood glucose reading sent to it by the continuous glucose meter.

Your doctor or health care team will help you manage your pump and insulin delivery. It's a good idea to carry a spare battery for your pump. Some physicians recommend that you carry backup equipment of a glucose monitor and insulin pen in case you have trouble with your pump or continuous glucose meter.

DIABETES LOGS

Keeping a record or log of your blood glucose test results, the food you eat, and the insulin you take can help you better control your diabetes. You might also want to include any changes to your schedule that could affect your glucose levels. Log sheets can be downloaded from the internet and printed. There are also apps that can help you keep track of your results.

No matter what method you use, record keeping may help you normalize your schedule. You'll be able to see at what times of the day your blood sugar is too high or too low and be able to make adjustments to help you maintain the proper balance.

TESTING DIABETES VALUES

When blood sugar levels are too high and insulin is too low, the cells aren't getting the fuel they need to function properly to maintain normal growth and development. Monitoring your blood sugar and ketones can ensure that you're controlling your diabetes. Two tests that tell you what your diabetes is doing at the moment are the finger stick test and the urine test.

FINGER STICK TEST

The finger stick test involves pricking your finger with a lancet to get a drop of blood. This blood sample is then inserted into a standard glucose monitor to determine your blood glucose level. Newer methods let you take a sample of blood from your arm or thigh.

Take readings before meals and at bedtime to see if your blood sugar is following a normal pattern throughout the day. This also helps determine if you and your health care team have found the proper balance between insulin, exercise, and diet to suit your individual needs. The ideal blood glucose level before a meal is between 80 to 130 mg/dl. Two hours after a meal the target number is less than 180 mg/dl. The normal blood glucose level for a person without diabetes is between 72 and 99 mg/dl before meals and less than 140 mg/dl two hours after eating.

Any change from your regular routine means that you need to test yourself so that you can modify your insulin intake to stay in balance. Test your blood glucose before you drive a car to avoid a hypoglycemic episode while on the road. Also, test your blood glucose when you wake up to see if the dawn phenomenon raises your values. Blood glucose testing is something you must do every day to ensure your health.

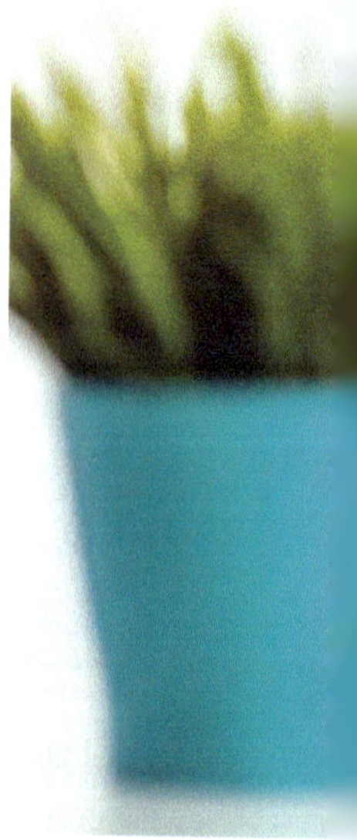

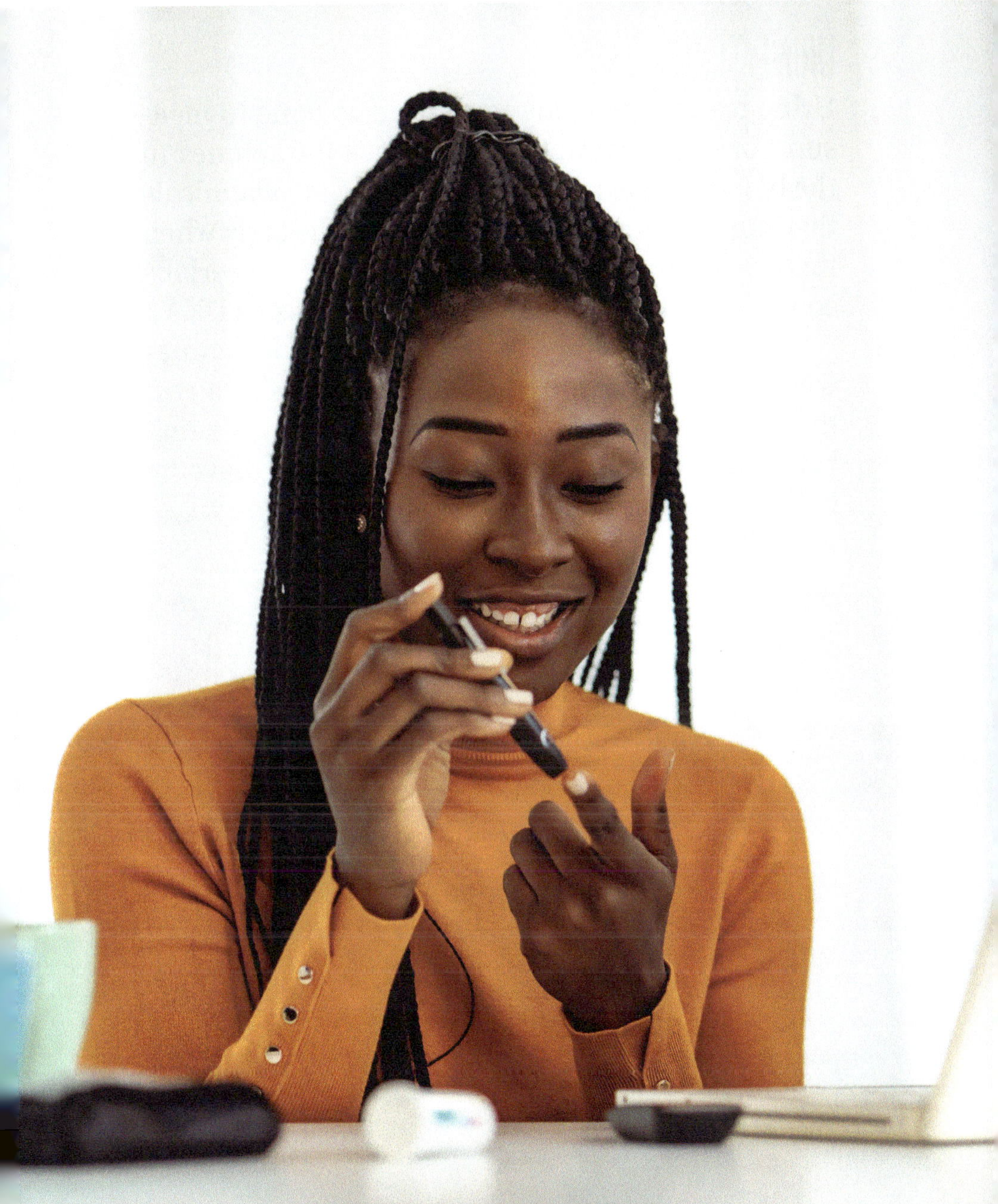

The finger stick test uses a lancing device to draw a drop of blood to test the glucose level in it.

URINE TESTS

Urine testing, by using test strips, is done to measure for ketones. Meters that check for ketones in the blood are also available. Ketones are chemicals that can accumulate to toxic levels in the body when there's not enough insulin. This can lead to a serious complication called diabetic ketoacidosis or DKA.

If you use insulin, you should test for ketones whenever you have two glucose readings in a row that are above 240 mg/dl. Both type 1 and type 2 diabetics should test whenever they get sick, have an infection, or experience extra stress.

AVOIDING DIABETIC KETOACIDOSIS (DKA)

Diabetic ketoacidosis, or DKA, is a dangerous complication of diabetes that can result in coma or death. It occurs when chemicals called ketones build up in the body because there's not enough insulin. Without insulin, glucose can't get into the cells and instead accumulates in the blood. Then the body burns fat instead of glucose for energy. This creates ketones, or chemicals, in the blood which then show up in urine.

Check for ketones when your blood glucose measures above 240 mg/dl. Also check for ketones when you're sick or have a noticeable change in diet. Ketones can be measured using a blood ketone meter, a breath ketone meter, or ketone strips that detect the chemicals in a urine sample.

Drinking water can flush out ketones. Symptoms of DKA include abdominal pain, confusion, fruity breath, nausea, rapid breathing, vomiting, and weakness. It requires medical treatment to replace fluids and electrolytes and to administer insulin.

MANAGING DIABETES VALUES

If your blood sugars are not within the desired range, you should recognize that the proportions between diet, insulin, and exercise have to be redesigned to achieve balance again. Also, the hormones associated with puberty can affect glucose levels. It's possible to experience a change in your blood sugar levels even if you're doing all the right things.

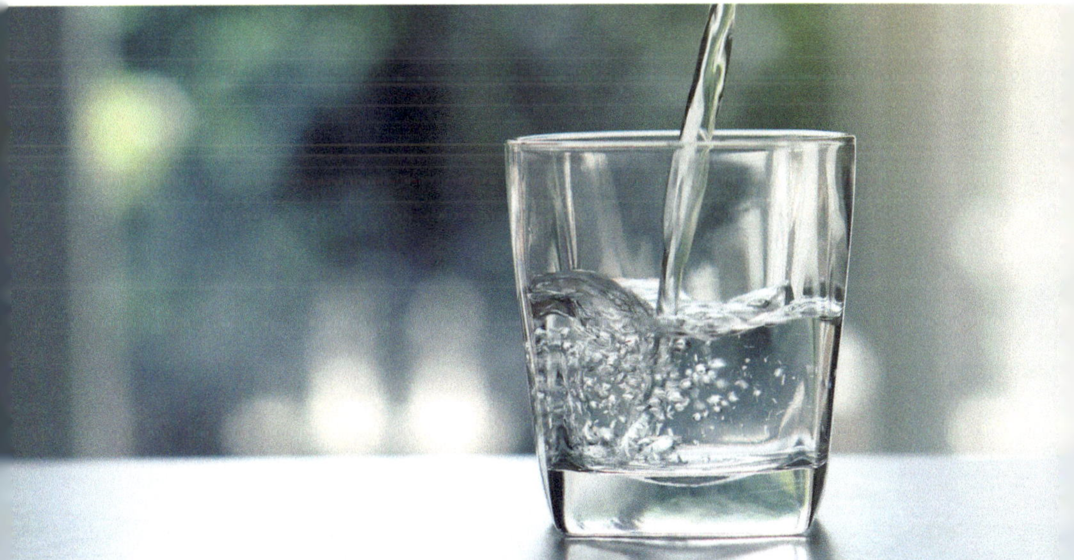

Drinking sugar-free liquids can help get rid of built-up ketones in the body. Water is the best option.

HYPOGLYCEMIA

Hypoglycemia, commonly called low blood sugar, happens when the blood glucose level drops below 70 mg/dl. It generally happens quickly and for reasons that you may be able to control, such as too much insulin, not eating enough food, skipping a snack or meal, or engaging in unexpected exercise.

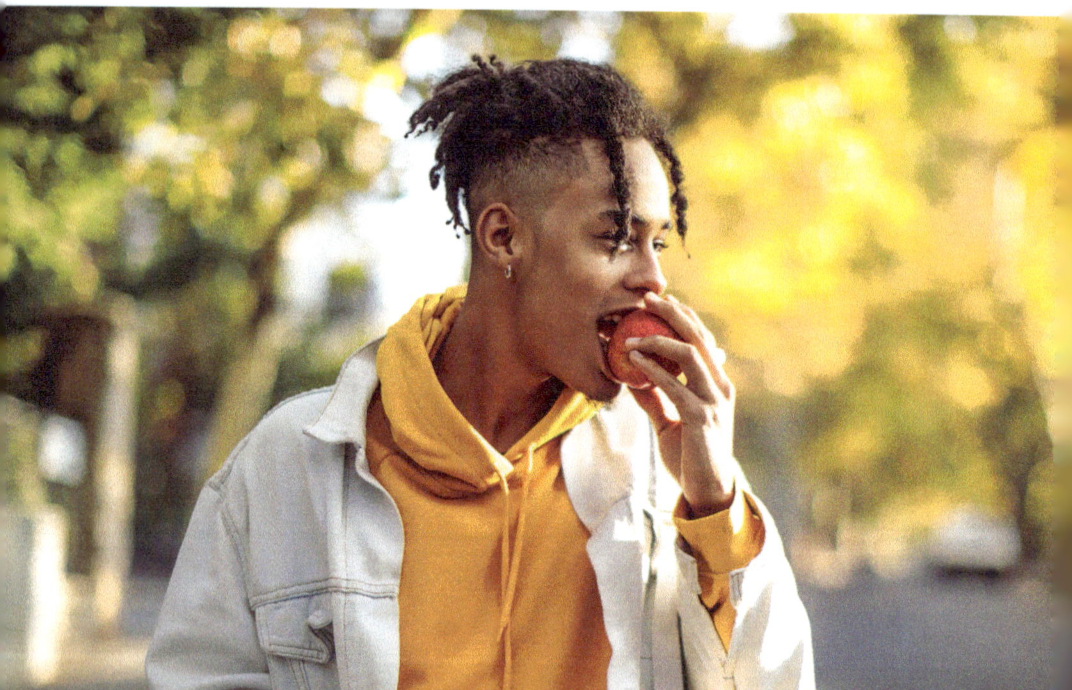

Apples usually only have a small effect on blood sugar levels. This means they're not likely to cause huge spikes in blood sugar. Several studies have also suggested that eating apples regularly may lower a person's risk of developing type 2 diabetes.

You can avoid hypoglycemia caused by insufficient food or missing a meal by carrying a snack with you. If you engage in extra exercise, check your glucose level as soon as you can. However, hypoglycemia may occur for no apparent reason.

If a person loses consciousness and can't ingest food to raise his or her glucose level, glucagon can be injected to raise the glucose level quickly. Family members and school personnel should be trained to be on the lookout for signs of hypoglycemia and know when and how to inject glucagon.

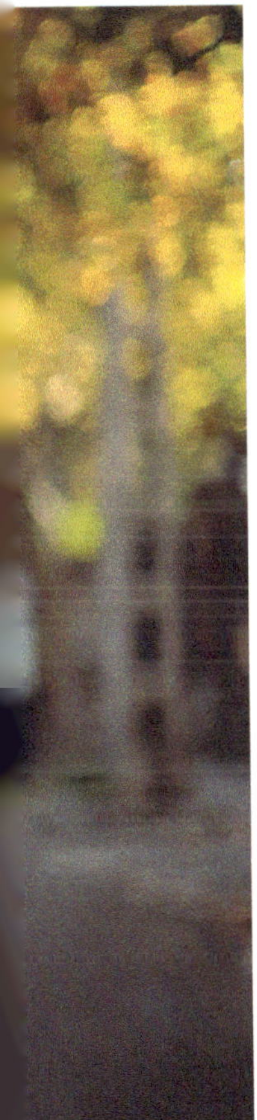

The symptoms of hypoglycemia are trembling, tingling lips, irritability, mood swings, sweating, hunger, fatigue, paleness, and loss of coordination. A person with hypoglycemia may also appear to be drunk. If you're with a friend who knows the symptoms, he or she will know you're suffering from hypoglycemia. But because you can't always be with people you know, hypoglycemia is a good reason to wear a medical alert bracelet. To treat hypoglycemia, you need a fast-acting sugar. There are several commercial products available that your doctor may recommend you keep close at hand. Hypoglycemia also can be treated with fruit juice, raisins, or hard candy. The benefits of commercial glucose tablets are that they work faster than candy and have fewer calories. Also, because the dosage is specific, you're less likely to push your blood glucose level up too high, which can happen with candy.

HYPERGLYCEMIA

Hyperglycemia is also called high blood sugar. It comes on slowly as a result of rising blood sugar levels. The symptoms are fatigue, extreme thirst, and frequent urination. When ketones begin to develop, you may feel nauseated and start to vomit, have stomach cramps, and your breath may smell sweet. Some of the causes of hyperglycemia, such as forgetting to take your insulin or eating too much of the wrong foods, can be prevented.

Hyperglycemia is treated by adjusting insulin intake. If you notice any of these symptoms, check your glucose levels immediately. Like hypoglycemia, hyperglycemia may occur no matter what you do. Hyperglycemia can develop into a coma if it's not caught in time. The best prevention is to monitor your glucose levels regularly, especially if you're not feeling well.

MAINTAINING TIGHT CONTROL OF DIABETES

Most people with diabetes follow a conventional approach to maintenance. That means they test a couple of times a day, use the same insulin dosage each day, and see their doctor about four times a year. Tight control means more of everything. It means testing, at the very least, four times a day and adjusting insulin dosages accordingly, which means injecting insulin several times a day or using an insulin pump.

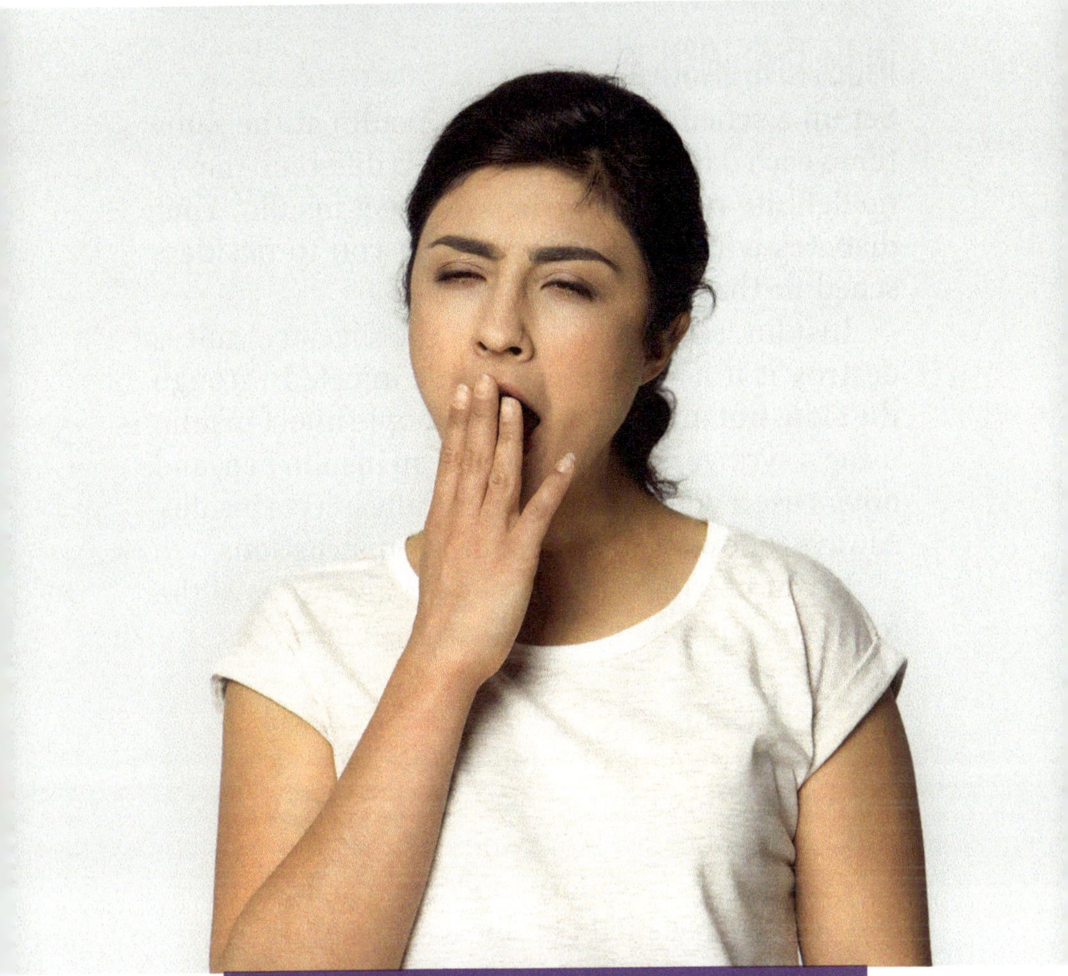

You might feel extra tired when experiencing hyperglycemia. If this happens, you should check your blood glucose levels right away.

If you have type 2 diabetes, the keys to tight control are diet and exercise. You might not have to monitor your blood glucose levels as frequently. With type 2 diabetes, your body does not use insulin efficiently, so glucose remains in your bloodstream. Exercise helps lower glucose levels.

INJECTING INSULIN

Set up a schedule to take your insulin at the same times each day. Because everyone is different, there's no definite rule about when to inject insulin. Your diabetes educator will work with you to decide a schedule that's right for you.

Insulin is injected because the digestive juices destroy it if it's taken orally. It's injected through the skin, not into a vein. Some people inject insulin using a syringe, some people use an insulin pen, and others use a pump that automatically injects insulin. Always follow the manufacturer's instructions.

If you use insulin, you should always have the following equipment readily accessible:

- Insulin
- Syringe, or pen and needle, or insulin pump
- Alcohol swab or wipe
- Emergency glucagon kit
- Glucose meter and test strips or continuous glucose monitor
- Medical identification card or bracelet

To administer your insulin properly, keep these rules in mind:

- Check the expiration date and never use outdated insulin. Don't buy more insulin than you can use before the expiration date.

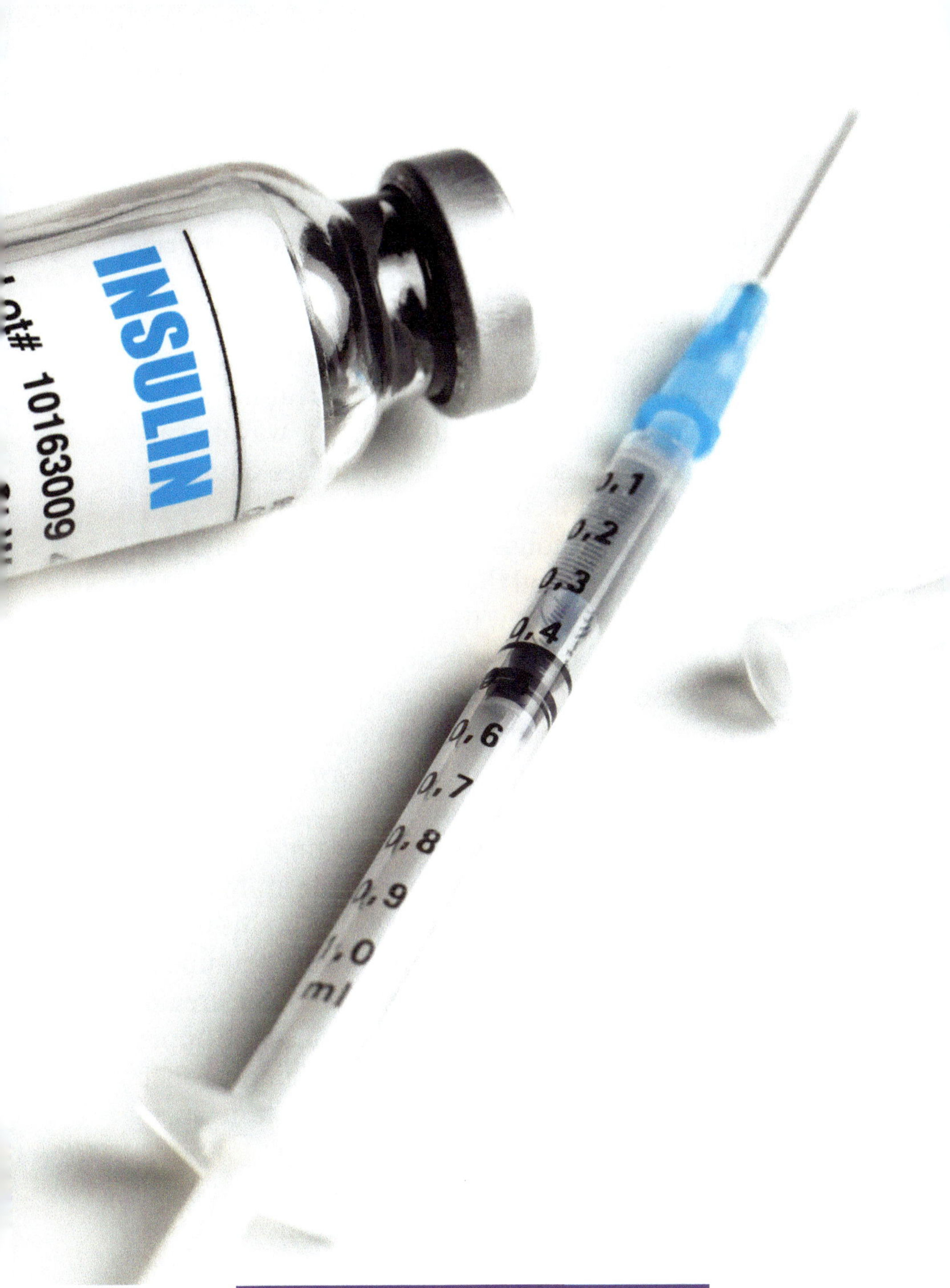

An older method of injecting insulin involves extracting the dose from a vial with a syringe.

• Store your supply of insulin in the refrigerator, but don't freeze it. (Researchers are working on developing an insulin that doesn't require refrigeration.) Keep the insulin you're currently using at room temperature and away from excessive cold or heat. Check with your doctor or pharmacist about the proper storage for your type of insulin.

• Make sure the insulin looks the way it's supposed to. Don't use the insulin if you see clumps of particles or crystals in it.

• Use an alcohol swab to wipe the top of the insulin vial or pen and the injection site. Don't reuse or share needles. Follow the dispensing instructions given by your diabetes educator or pharmacist.

• Know the name or type of insulin you use, the company that makes it, the concentration, and the dosage. Keep a copy of this information in your wallet or store it on your phone.

• Rotate the injection site each time to prevent little lumps, called lipodystrophies, from forming. To inject insulin, pinch a section of skin, insert the needle, and then release the skin while you inject. Some places commonly used are the outer area of the upper arm, just below the hip bone in the upper buttock, above and below the waist avoiding a 2-inch circle around the navel, and the middle front of the thigh.

• When you're injecting insulin just before physical activity, don't inject it into the area you will be using the most. For example, if you're going to be running, don't inject insulin into your leg. It will absorb much faster than you're used to.

TYPE 2 DIABETES MEDICATION

The most common therapy for people with type 2 diabetes is diet and exercise. For some people, however, diet and exercise are insufficient to control their blood glucose levels. Those patients are given oral medications. There are several categories of these medications, which may be prescribed alone, in combination with other drugs, or with insulin. Your doctor and your health care team can help you determine which drug or drugs are best for you. Each medication has different side effects. One drug may be more effective for you than another.

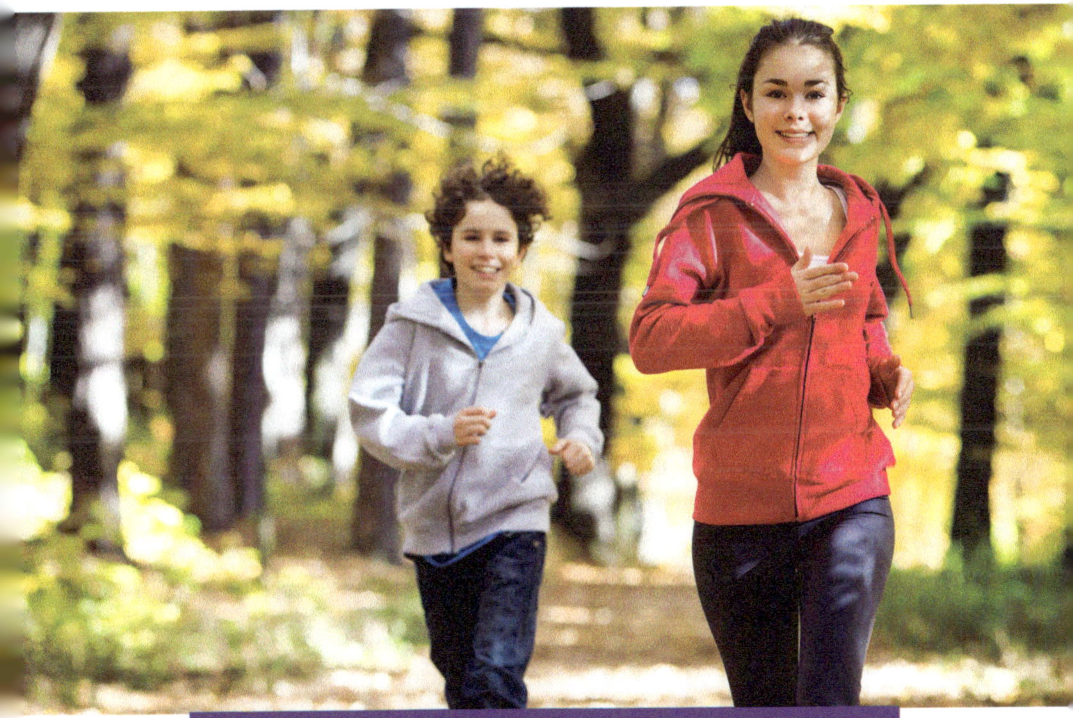

Running and jogging are great forms of exercise. Paired with a healthy diet, exercising regularly can be a great way to manage type 2 diabetes.

CHAPTER 5

STAYING HEALTHY WITH DIABETES

Advances in medical science have allowed people with diabetes to live long and healthy lives. There's still no cure, and diabetics still face an increased risk for other health issues over a period of time. Diabetes can cause problems with your eyes, kidneys, heart, feet, skin, and nerves. What you do now to take care of yourself can affect your future. Keeping yourself healthy will decrease your risk of developing some of these complications.

EYES

People with diabetes need to take extra care of their eyes by having regular eye exams. A serious eye disease is diabetic retinopathy. This occurs when the small vessels of the retina become weak or swell, which results in leakage of blood. Some blood vessels close and new ones grow and interfere with vision. In type 1 diabetes, blurry vision can be a symptom of hypoglycemia or hyperglycemia, not necessarily eye disease. Good control of blood glucose is the key to preventing diabetic retinopathy. Researchers have found that keeping your blood pressure under control also can reduce the risk of this complication.

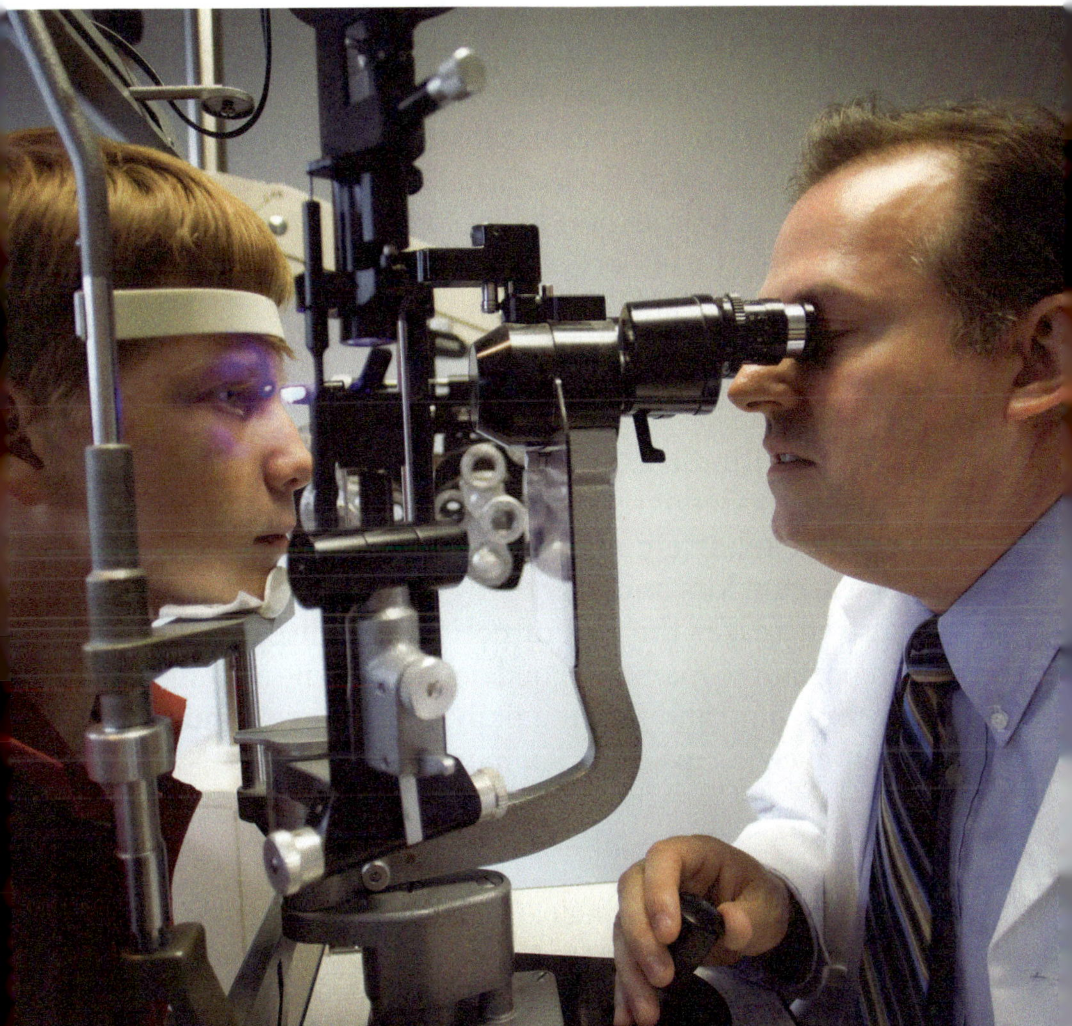

Regular eye exams are important to screen for eye diseases that can be caused by high blood glucose.

You can have diabetic retinopathy and still have good vision. Fortunately, there are treatments to prevent blindness in people diagnosed with diabetic retinopathy. Focal laser treatment can reduce the loss of vision in the early stages. People with diabetes are also at greater risk for cataracts (a condition in which the lens clouds up and looks milky) and glaucoma (a condition caused by increased pressure in the eye) which can cause loss of vision over time.

All of these eye diseases can be treated if detected early enough by an ophthalmologist or retinologist. Therefore, it's important that an eye specialist is a part of your health care team.

TEETH

People with diabetes are more prone to gum disease or periodontal disease if their glucose levels are not relatively stable. Periodontal disease can cause gum loss and eventually tooth loss. Smoking also increases the risk of periodontal disease. It's important to maintain good dental hygiene at home by brushing and flossing daily and to have regular dental checkups every six months.

KIDNEYS

Diabetes is the leading cause of kidney disease and can cause tissue damage to the organs over a period of time. This damage is called diabetic nephropathy and can lead to end-stage renal disease. End-stage renal disease occurs when a person's kidneys have

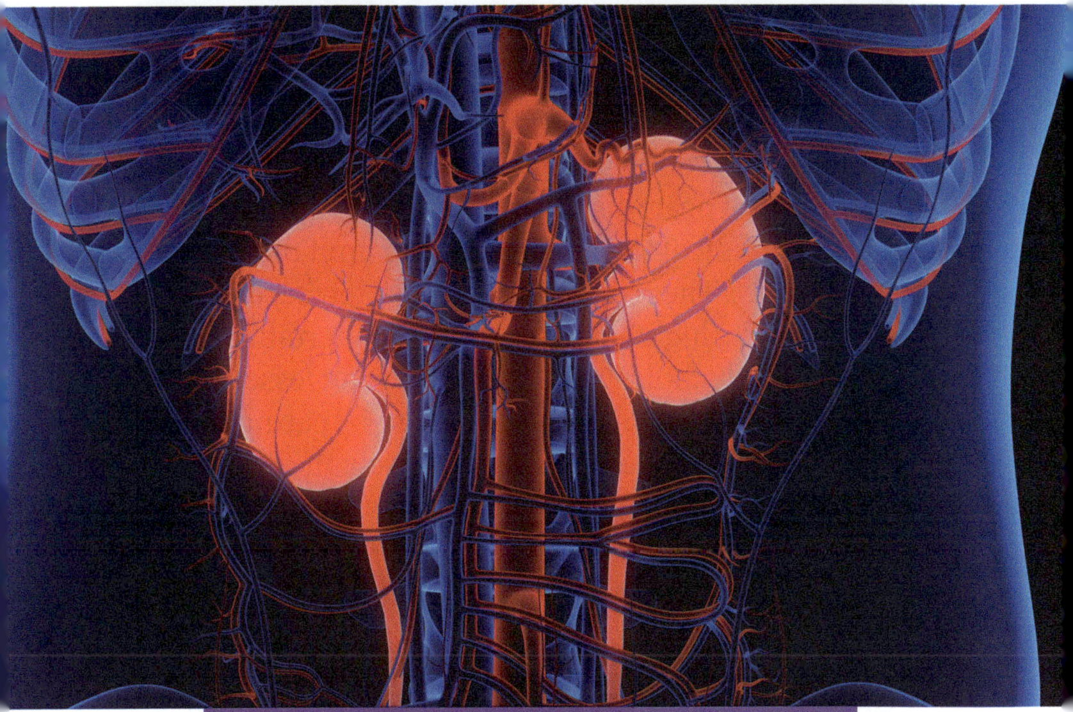

Most people are born with two kidneys, shown here in red. They're shaped a bit like beans and are located on either side of the spine.

lost their ability to function. A person with end-stage renal disease needs to have kidney dialysis or a kidney transplant to stay alive. High blood pressure increases the chances of developing this disease. If you have type 2 diabetes and smoke cigarettes or have high cholesterol levels, you further increase your risk for renal disease. Controlling your blood sugar and your blood pressure can prevent or delay kidney complications. In addition, any urinary tract infection should be treated immediately. Your doctor should perform a urinalysis every year to determine the potential for this disease.

HEART

People with diabetes face an increased risk of developing heart problems. High glucose levels contribute to the risk of heart disease by increasing the potential for hardening of the arteries, which limit blood flow to the heart. The risk of heart disease increases if you smoke, have high blood pressure, use certain drugs, or have high cholesterol levels. You can lessen your chances of developing heart disease by eating a balanced diet, maintaining a healthy weight, exercising regularly, and keeping your diabetes under control.

NERVOUS SYSTEM

Diabetes can cause changes in the nervous system causing neuropathy. These changes may feel like a tingling or buzzing. Hands and feet may become numb. You may not be able to tell the difference between hot and cold, and you may not notice small cuts at first. As with most other diabetes complications, the risk for diabetic neuropathy increases if you have poor blood glucose control, smoke, drink alcohol, or have high blood pressure.

LEGS AND FEET

It's important to take care of your legs and feet. Diabetes can damage the nerves and cause problems with blood flow in these areas. Smoking cigarettes increases the risk of damage to the nerves in the feet. If you have neuropathy in your legs or feet, you may not be able to feel a cut or sore. Check your feet daily, dry between your toes, and wear water shoes (not flip flops or sandals) at the beach or pool. Infections and poor blood flow are the major cause for amputations in diabetics.

SKIN

If your diabetes is not properly controlled, you may become dehydrated, causing your skin to become dry and itchy. Try using a lanolin-based cream or moisturizer. If you find the skin between your toes getting dry and cracked, consult your doctor. High blood glucose levels interfere with the action of bacteria-fighting cells, making diabetics more prone to skin infections. If you get a sore or a cut anywhere, treat it immediately. If it doesn't heal readily, you may need your doctor to prescribe an antibiotic.

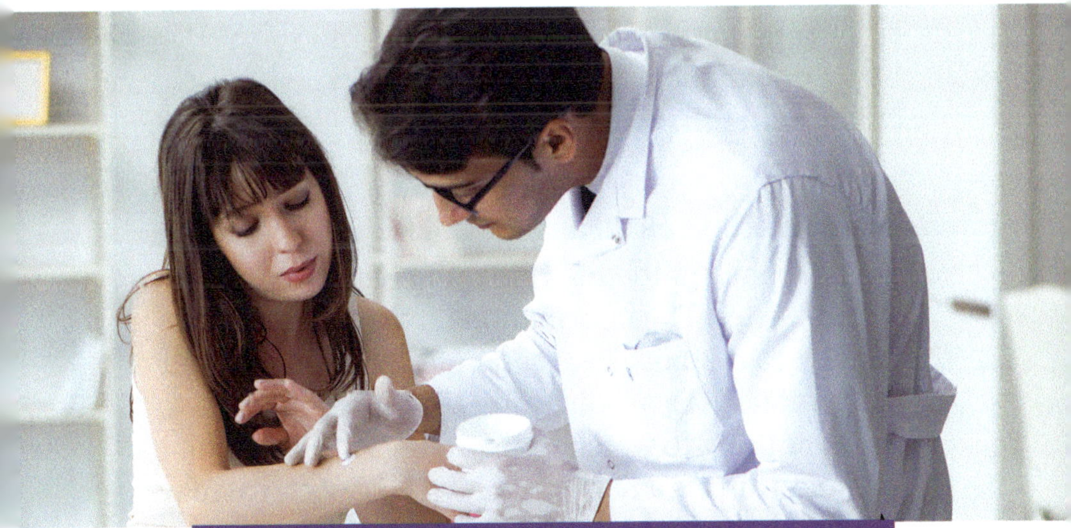

A doctor may be able to prescribe special topical creams to treat painful skin conditions that may happen as a result of diabetes or its symptoms.

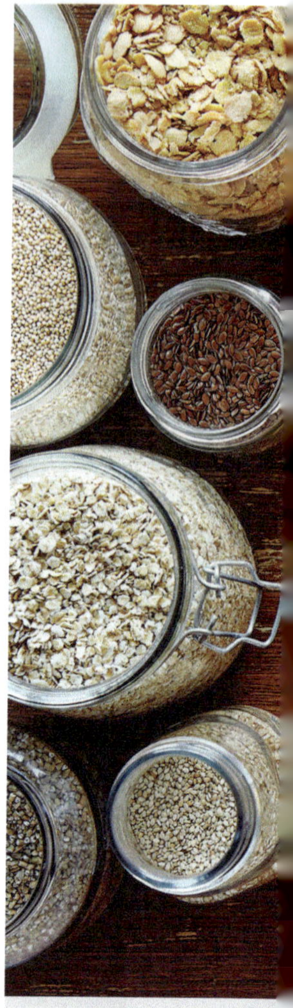

DIABETES AND DIET

The fundamental key to good health is a good diet. This is especially true for people with diabetes. Although you can still eat the things you like, you must do so in moderation. Part of everything you eat is turned into glucose. Because your body doesn't produce or use insulin effectively, you must carefully balance the amount of glucose you have and the amount of insulin you take. If you have type 2 diabetes, diet may be your main means of controlling the disease.

The purpose of a healthier diet in a person with diabetes is to control the blood glucose level. If you start taking care of your body now, you lessen the risks of diabetic complications later in life. Your diabetes educator can help create a diet that works for you.

CHECKING FOOD LABELS

Food labeling guidelines are quite helpful to people with diabetes. The information on the nutrition facts panel on a food package can help you monitor your daily intake of carbohydrates, proteins, and fats. Another thing to watch for is the serving size. What you may think is a normal-size serving of cereal may actually be twice the product's serving size. Learn to weigh and measure your foods, especially carbo-

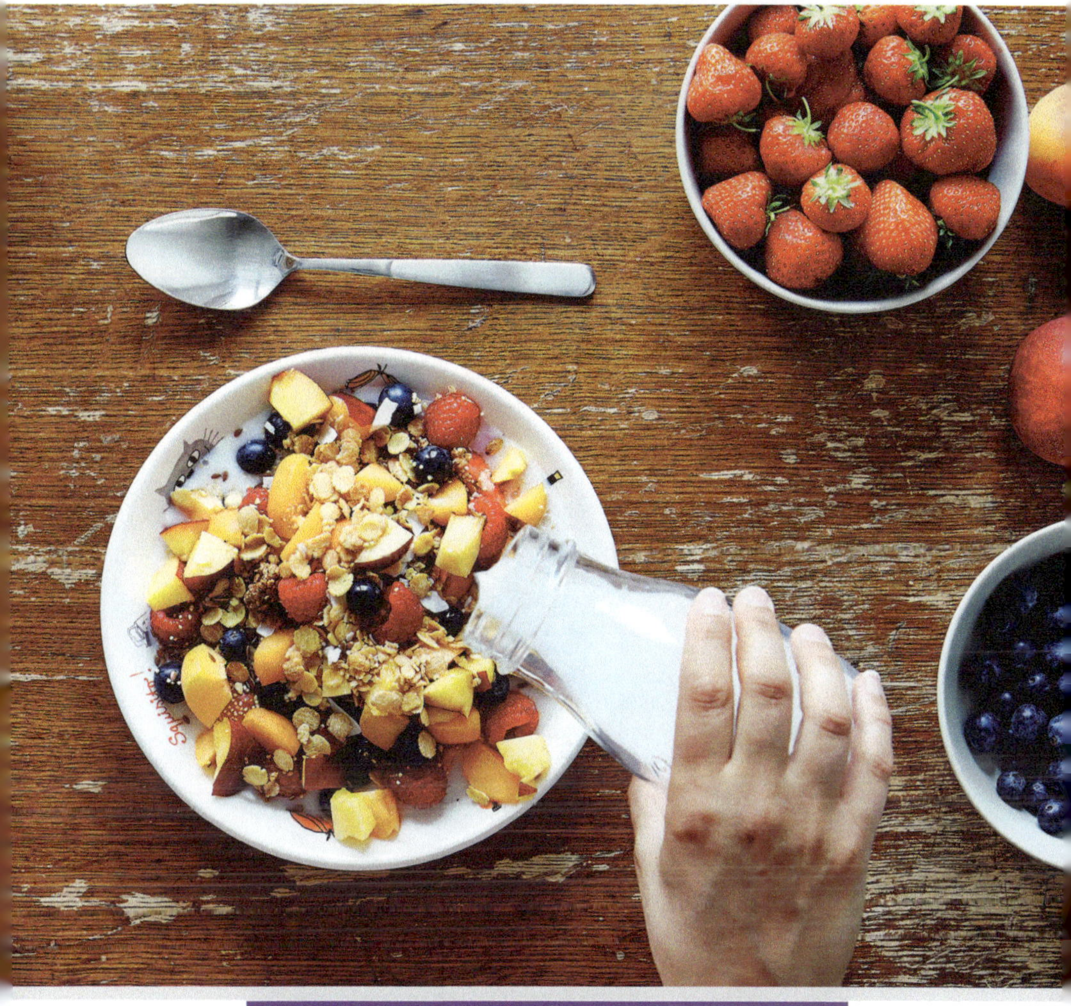

The nutrition facts panel on a food package label can help to determine the amount of insulin required for a serving size.

hydrates. Also, learn the difference between simple and complex carbohydrates and how they raise blood sugar. Teens tend to need a higher caloric intake. The key is to consume nutritious foods rather than calories that have no nutritional value.

DIABETIC ALERT DOGS (DADS)

You've probably heard of or seen a guide dog helping a blind person. There are different kinds of Medical Alert Dogs that assist people with their disabilities. This includes Diabetic Alert Dogs, or DADs, that are trained just to help diabetics. They alert their diabetic human before they're about to experience hypoglycemia (low

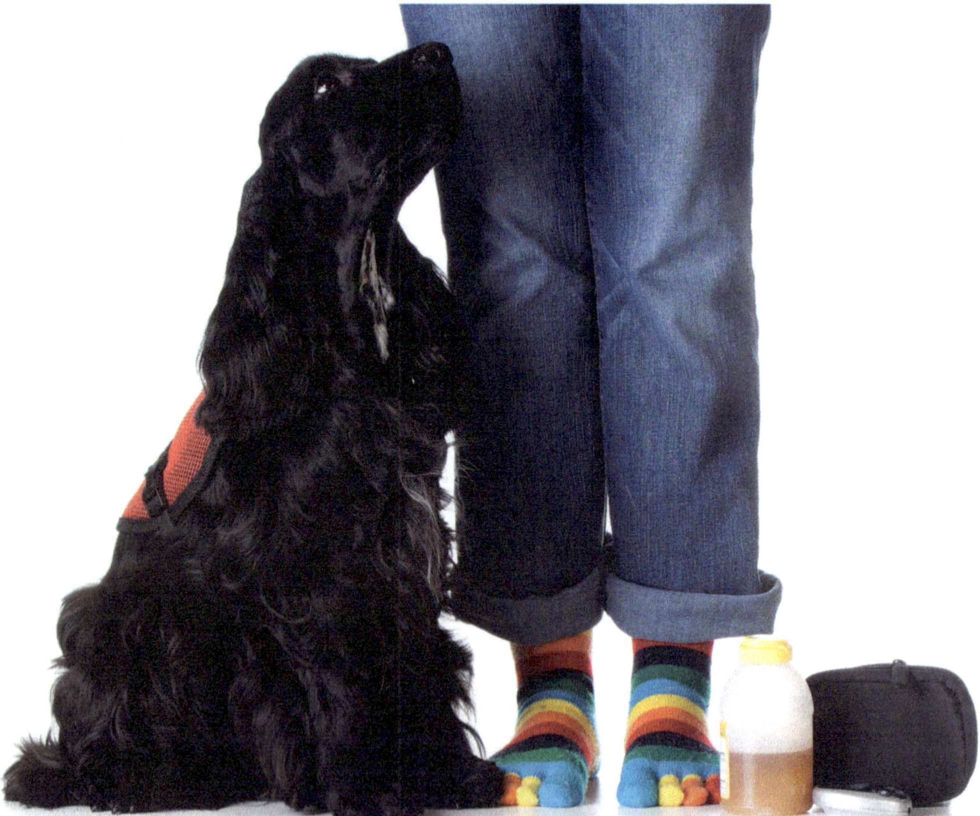

A diabetic alert dog can sense a shift to dangerous blood glucose levels in a person with diabetes.

blood glucose) or hyperglycemia (high blood glucose). This can help the diabetic patient take the necessary steps to avoid blood sugar values that could pose a serious health risk.

When a person with diabetes is about to have dangerously low or high blood sugar, a chemical shift occurs in their body. This shift gives off a smell that only a trained DAD can sense. Depending on how they were trained, there are different ways that a DAD can alert their diabetic human. DADs also provide emotional comfort and support to their human as they manage their diabetes.

It's important to get a DAD through an accredited organization so that your dog is properly trained. It can take six months to a year to get a DAD and can cost a few thousand dollars.

DIABETES AND EXERCISE

Regular exercise helps maintain your weight, tone your muscles, and control your insulin levels. If you take insulin, you must learn to recognize that different types of activities use up different calorie values. You need this information so that you can adjust your food intake accordingly.

Excessive exercise can leave you with too little blood glucose. You should be prepared for this by carrying a fast-acting sugar food or glucose tablets. Test your blood sugar before you exercise; if it's low, you may have to raise it. If you participate in after-school sports and the coach calls for that extra practice, be prepared by bringing a fast sugar food with you. If you begin to experience the symptoms of

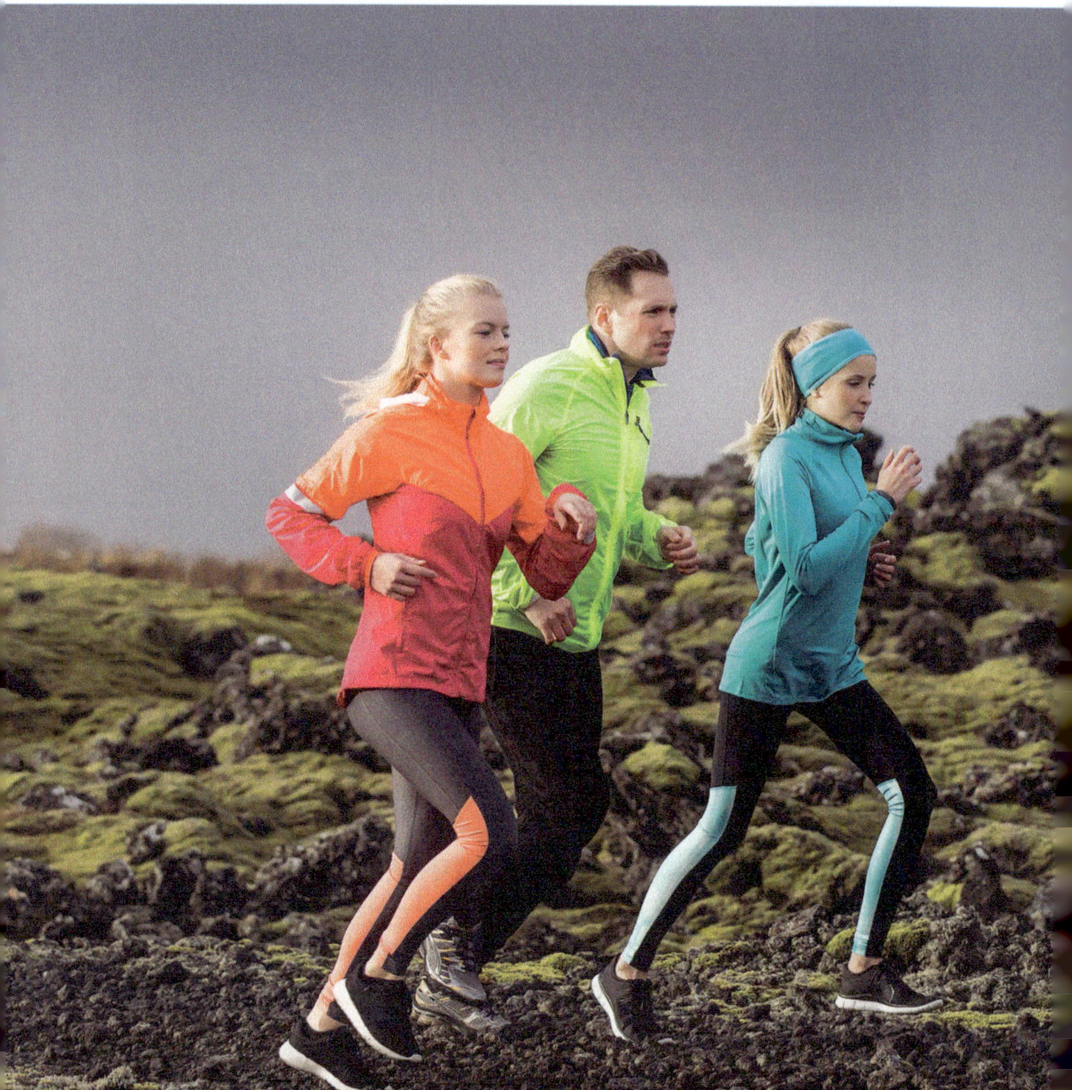

Exercise helps people with diabetes keep healthy, but they must balance the type of activity with the right amount of insulin.

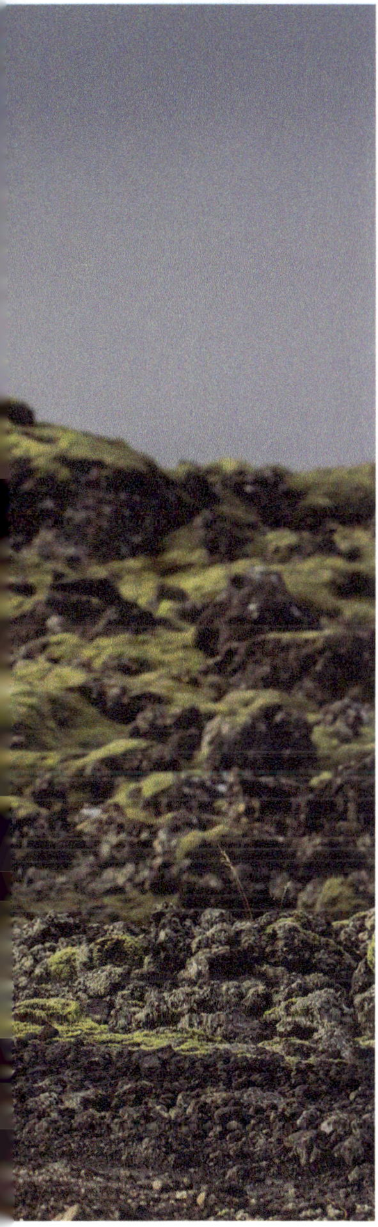

low blood sugar, stop exercising and take care of yourself immediately. It's also a good idea to have a high-carbohydrate snack before you begin any exercise or sports. If you're using a pump, check with your doctor if you should reduce your basal insulin before any exercise or sports.

Remember that exercise must be balanced with insulin. Exercise burns up extra glucose in the blood when there is a sufficient supply of insulin in the body. If insulin is not balanced with exercise, you may find your glucose levels rising after a workout. If you find that exercise raises your blood sugar levels, you may have to take more insulin or forgo that extra workout and wait until your glucose level falls. With a little practice, you'll be able to find the right balance of exercise and insulin that'll work for you.

CHAPTER 6

LIVING WITH DIABETES

Growing up is about learning new things and having new experiences. Diabetes shouldn't hold you back from experiencing new things. It's wise, however, to consider how certain experiences or events could affect your diabetes and possibly endanger your health.

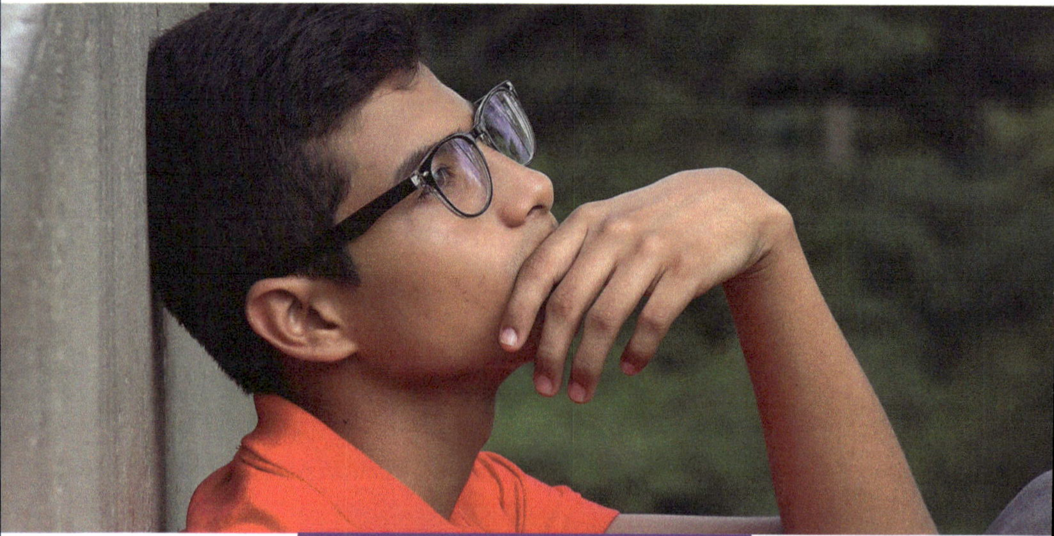

People with diabetes need to think about how some experiences might affect their disease.

ALCOHOL

Alcohol can be dangerous for diabetics because it interferes with blood sugar levels. This is because your liver can't process alcohol and release glucose at the same time. Many diabetes medicines warn that mixing alcohol with medication could cause serious problems. Another thing to remember is that a person experiencing hypoglycemia can appear to be drunk to others, thus delaying help or medical assistance.

DRUGS

Drugs are dangerous for people without diabetes and can pose serious health consequences. The use of drugs can result in poor regulation of blood glucose levels, weight gain, and the development of complications. Also, it's not easy to remember to monitor your blood glucose levels if you're high on drugs.

TOBACCO

You already know about the dangers of smoking for people without diabetes. For people with diabetes, the dangers are even greater. Smoking can lead to long-term complications and premature death. Smoking narrows the blood vessels and decreases circulation to the limbs, sometimes resulting in limb amputations in diabetics.

BODY PIERCINGS AND TATTOOS

Body piercing involves creating a hole in your body somewhere and inserting jewelry. Many people have their ears pierced. However, piercing your earlobe is not the same as piercing another part of your anatomy. Healing can take several weeks to several months with a constant chance of serious infection and secondary infection (an infection in another area caused by the first infection).

Tattooing is a process where pigment is injected under the skin to produce permanent designs. Anyone getting a tattoo must be certain that they're in a clean, antiseptic environment and that the tattoo artist is a skilled professional. Having diabetes means your immune system is not always as strong as someone who doesn't have diabetes. Make certain you keep the tattoo clean and continue to monitor your glucose levels closely.

DIABETES AND TRAVEL

Diabetes should not interfere with any travel, but you need to plan ahead. Make certain you have enough medication with you. Don't pack it in a suitcase that might get lost. Use a travel cooler to store insulin that you'll use later in your trip. Keep it cool but not frozen. Carry a copy of any prescriptions you may need. Also, carry fast-acting sugar food or glucose tablets or glucose gel packets with you. If you cross time zones, remember to adjust your medication accordingly. Wear a medical alert bracelet or medallion. There are many stylish options from which to choose.

If you travel by plane, it's important to follow the guidelines of the Transportation Security Administration (TSA) for packing and taking your diabetic equipment and supplies through the screening checkpoints. You can contact the TSA before your flight to make the check-in process easier. If you travel abroad, check the laws in each country regarding carrying prescription drugs. You can read about the experiences of people with diabetes traveling worldwide on websites and blogs on the internet.

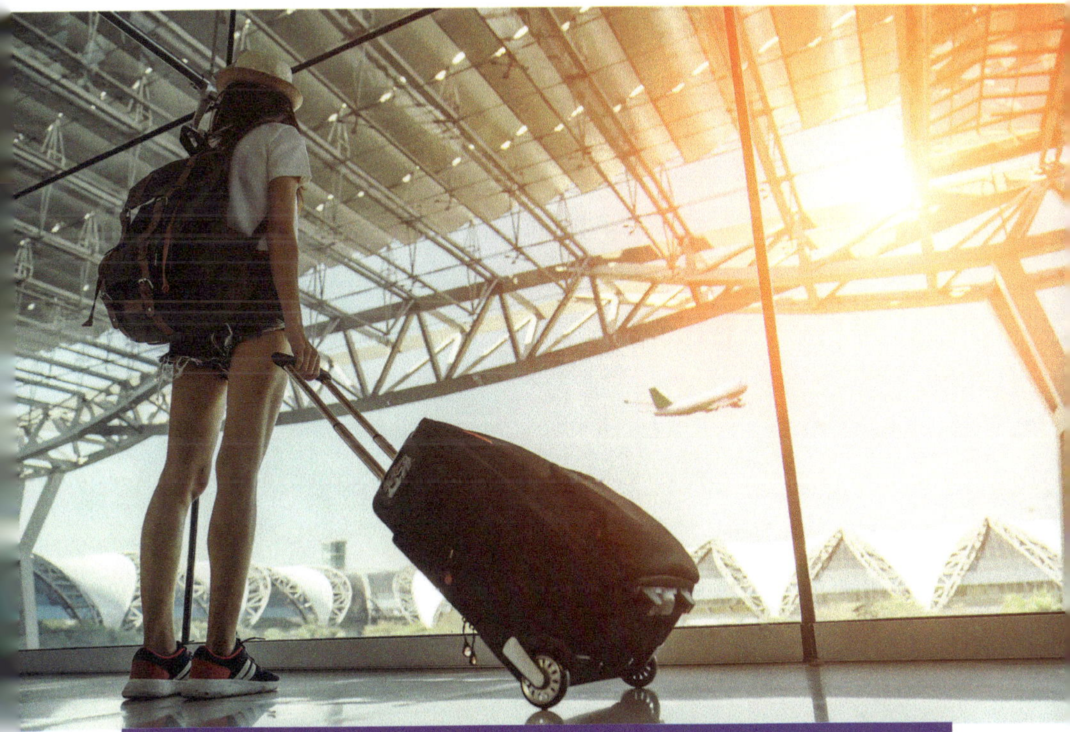

Make sure to read the TSA's rules about packing diabetes medication before you go to the airport. This can make for a smoother experience when you go through security.

CAMPS FOR PEOPLE WITH DIABETES

There are many summer camps for young people with diabetes. These camps are a great place to make friends with people who already understand most of what you're going through and who can share similar experiences with you. At these camps, you can learn more about diabetes, how to maintain control of it, and grow confident and independent in managing it. Because all of the campers, and many of the staff, at these camps have diabetes, everyone can be more open with each other. Sometimes it just feels good to be able to relax and have fun and not have to explain about having diabetes.

Remember to choose a camp that belongs to the Diabetes Education & Camping Association. They're usually affiliated with a diabetes treatment center whose staff volunteer or work with the campers.

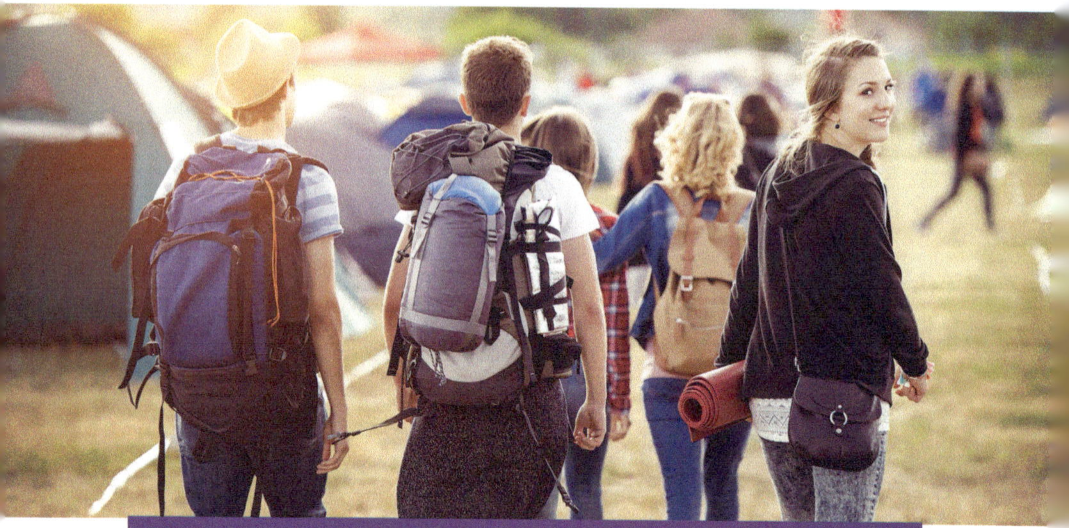

Camp can be a fun experience for anyone. When you go to a camp specifically for people with diabetes, you don't have to worry about feeling different or like you're the only one taking breaks from activities to monitor your glucose levels.

DIABETES IN MALES

Diabetes in males can cause sexual dysfunction or impotence, the inability to maintain an erection. You increase your risk of developing this complication if you smoke, drink alcoholic beverages, or don't keep your blood glucose levels under control. Out-of-control diabetes also can inhibit growth.

DIABETES IN FEMALES

Menstruation can raise and lower your blood glucose levels. Also, it's common for young women to use larger amounts of insulin at night during the week before their period. Therefore, it's important to follow your glucose level testing schedules. Consult your health care team if your blood glucose levels fluctuate greatly.

Women have to be watchful for yeast infections. Symptoms are vaginal itching and a white discharge. Yeast infections are caused by a fungus, *Candida albicans*, which flourishes on high blood glucose and moisture. Wear cotton underwear to decrease moisture. As always, the first line of defense is to keep your diabetes under control.

TYPE 2 DIABETES AND WEIGHT LOSS

If you're overweight and have been diagnosed with type 2 diabetes, you need to monitor your calorie and fat intake. Your health care team can help you to develop a diet and exercise plan that you can stick to. Try to stay away from fast food and soda. Fast food is usually high in carbohydrates and soda is high in empty calories. Remember that this is your greatest growth period, and out-of-control diabetes can inhibit growth.

DIABETES AND ILLNESS

When you're sick with the flu, a cold, or anything else, it's important to keep up with testing your blood glucose and administering insulin. Good control of your diabetes is necessary for the body to heal and avoid complications. Check with your doctor or health care team on how any medicines you take, such as acetaminophen or ibuprofen, might affect your blood glucose levels and insulin requirements. Consider getting a flu shot every year. People with and without diabetes can die from complications of the flu. The flu is a viral respiratory infection that can lead to pneumonia. High blood glucose levels impair the body's ability to fight infection.

DIABETES AND YOUR RIGHTS

You have a right to be treated with respect when your doctor and your health care team talks with you about diabetes and your care. They shouldn't lecture or yell at you. If any member of your health care team treats you with disrespect or doesn't clearly explain things, speak up. Managing your diabetes is a team effort, and you're the most important member of the team.

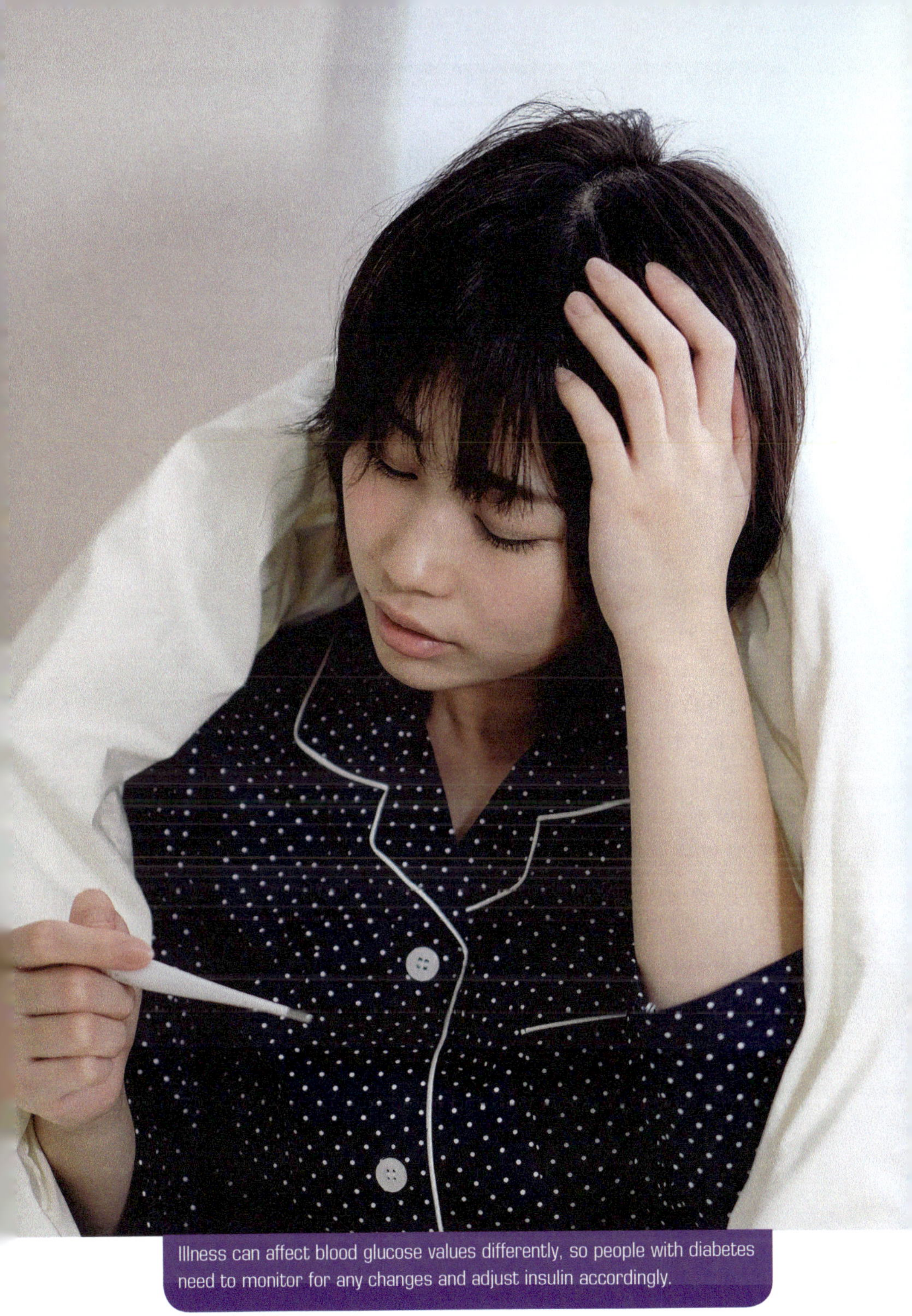

Illness can affect blood glucose values differently, so people with diabetes need to monitor for any changes and adjust insulin accordingly.

You have a right to have all procedures, tests, and medications explained to you in language you can understand. Ask the doctor to explain any information that isn't clear. After all, you are the one most responsible for managing your diabetes.

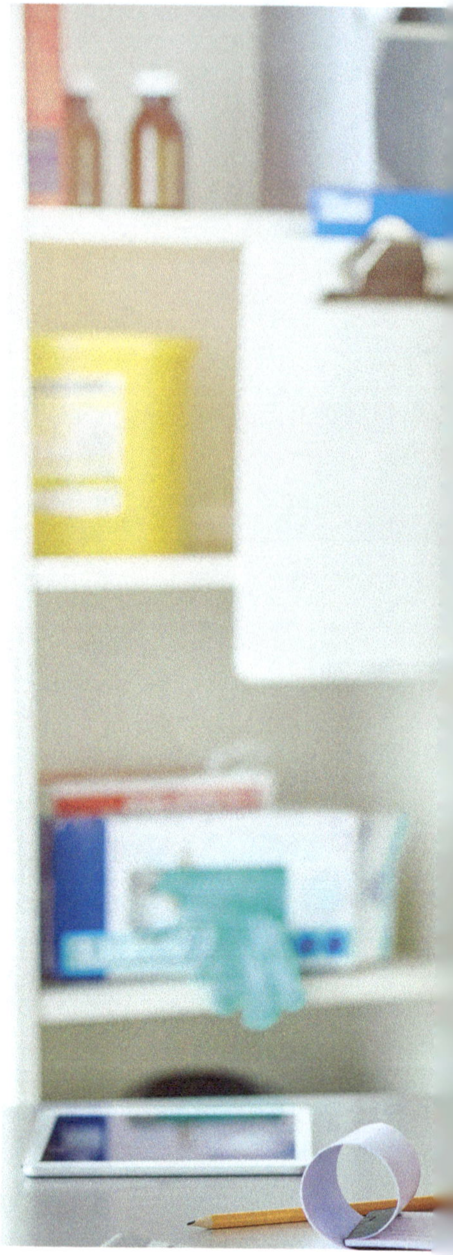

You have a right to know about the variety of treatments available. Some doctors are partial to certain kinds of treatment. If you've heard about a new treatment, you have a right to expect your doctor to discuss it with you.

You have a right to privacy. There may be some things you want to discuss with your health care team privately. You may have questions about birth control, drugs, or how diabetes may affect your sex life in the future. Don't assume that confidentiality is the rule. You're still considered a minor and under your parents' protection.

Just as you have a right to expect certain things from

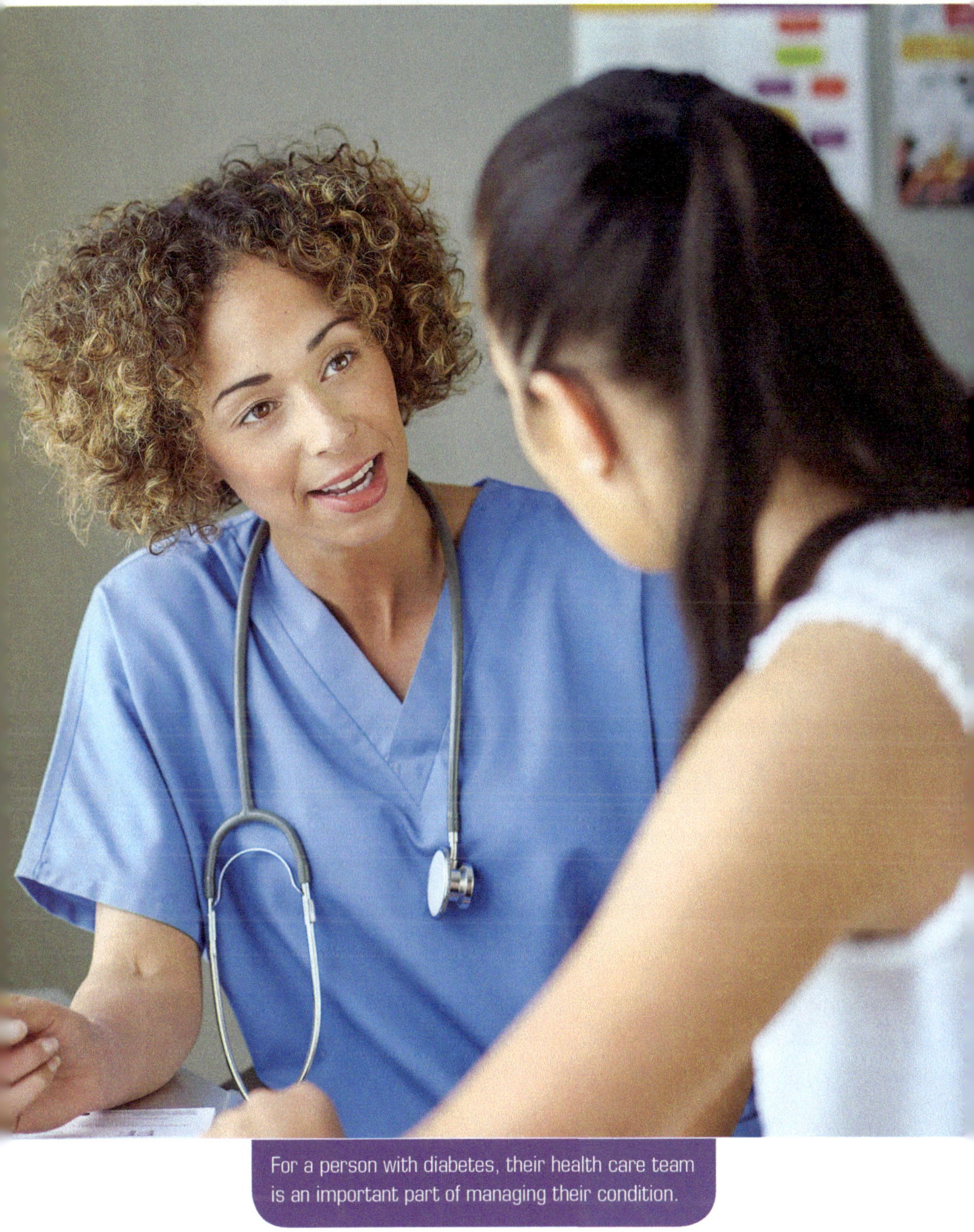

For a person with diabetes, their health care team is an important part of managing their condition.

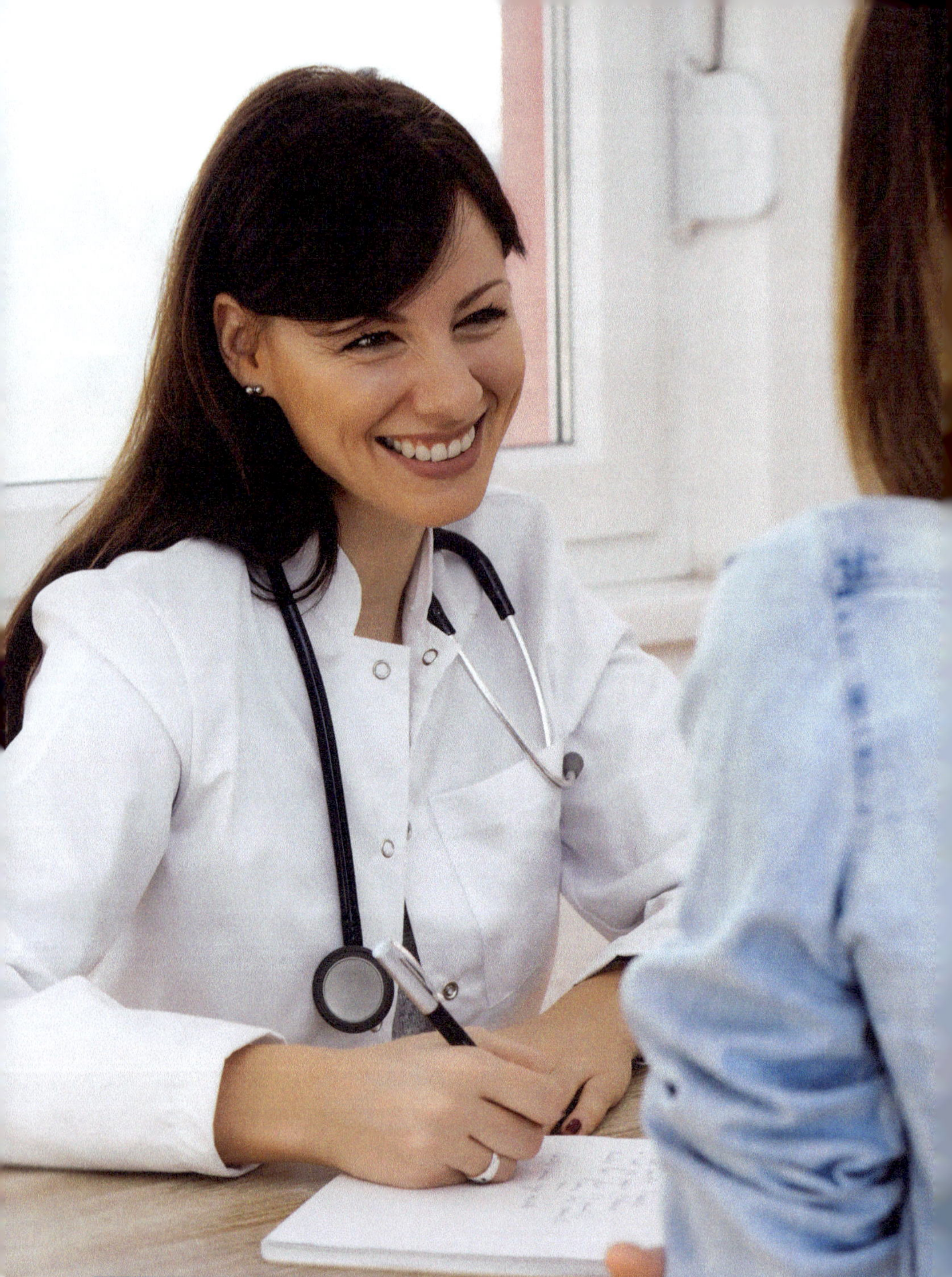

It's important to get along with your doctors, especially when you have a condition, such as diabetes, that requires you to communicate closely with your health care team.

your health care team, they have a right to expect certain things from you. They have a right to expect you to be honest about your testing habits, record keeping, eating habits, and exercise. Your honesty will guide them and you toward managing your diabetes as well as possible.

If you find that you and your health care team don't get along for any reason or because your personalities just don't fit together, ask your parents to find another doctor. It's important to get along with your health care team. You must feel comfortable with them and be able to trust their judgments and opinions.

You have a right to be accepted by teachers and classmates. In return, the school and your teachers have a right to expect you to provide them with the information necessary to help them care for you in the event of an emergency. You have a right to check your blood glucose and inject your insulin as needed.

CHAPTER 7

ADVANCES IN DIABETES MANAGEMENT

Diabetes is a chronic disease that so far has no known cure. The way diabetes affects your future depends on how well you take care of yourself today. There are very few limitations on what you can do or who you can become if you control your diabetes. Diabetes shouldn't control you.

Some career choices might be limited or require a medical certificate for people with insulin-dependent diabetes. The possibility of a hypoglycemic event or another complication could pose a danger for the employee, coworkers, or other people. Restrictions might apply to people with diabetes operating heavy machinery and driving or flying commercial vehicles. Employment might be considered on a case-by-case basis and employers are urged to take each person as an individual. For most jobs, you aren't required to tell an employer that you have diabetes. The Americans with Disabilities Act of 1992 protects employees from discrimination.

SUCCESSFUL PEOPLE WITH DIABETES

Diabetes shouldn't hold you back from pursuing your dreams and achieving your goals. Many well-known people with diabetes haven't let the disease hold them back from success. They include people from all walks of life and professions.

Entertainer Nick Jonas was diagnosed with type 1 diabetes when he was 13 years old. In 2015, Jonas founded Beyond Type 1, an organization that brings awareness to what it's like to live with diabetes.

(continued on next page)

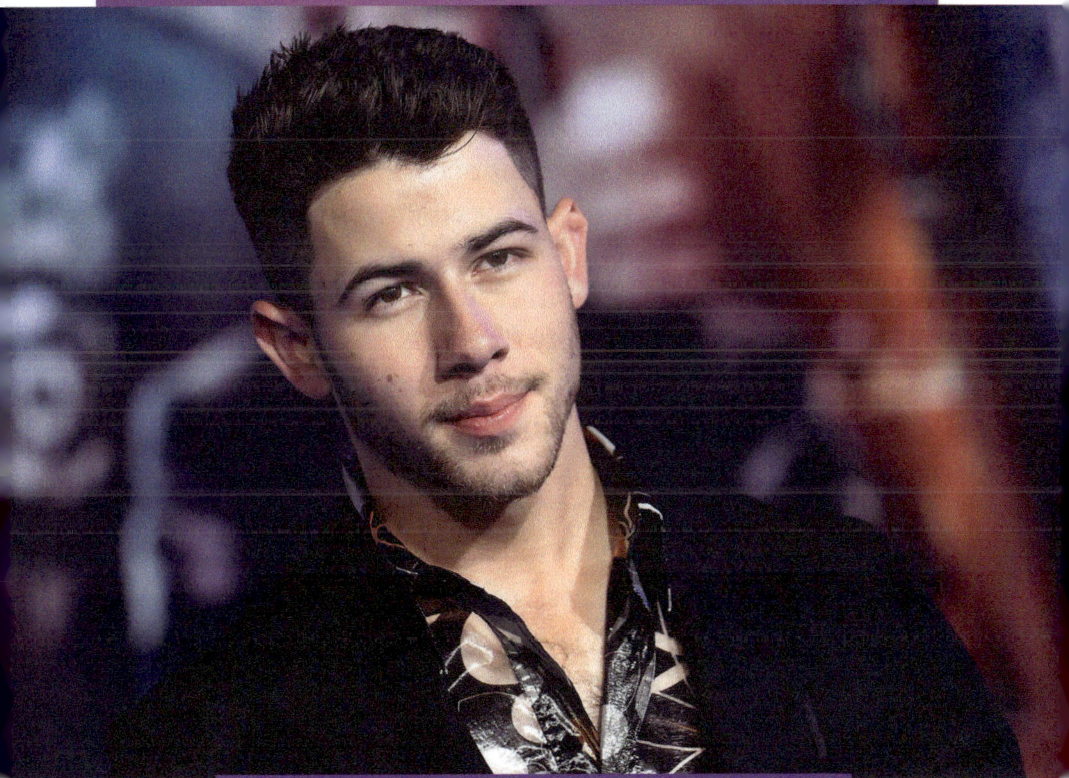

Nick Jonas hasn't let diabetes stop him from working in different areas of the entertainment field and founding Beyond Type 1.

(continued from previous page)

George Lucas, the director of Star Wars, found out he had type 2 diabetes when he was a young adult. U.S. Supreme Court Judge Sonia Sotomayor has had type 1 diabetes since age seven. Adam Duvall didn't let diabetes prevent him from playing major league baseball. Several young people with diabetes are known on social media for sharing how they manage their condition. On TikTok, Beth McDaniel and Eileen Watson are called the Diabetic Duo and have more than 21,000 followers. Diabetic Danica shares videos with her nearly 40,000 YouTube subscribers on various topics on living with type 1 diabetes.

ADVANCES IN DIABETES RESEARCH

In the past few years, there have been many breakthrough advances in how diabetes is monitored and treated. Scientists and doctors continue to research more effective and easier ways to measure blood glucose and deliver insulin. Researchers also have learned more about how diabetes affects the body and how to avoid complications.

More accurate ways to determine blood glucose are being developed. Currently, measuring blood glucose relies on an enzyme that can change. Instead, scientists are looking at using a molecule that stays stable for a longer period of time.

It's known that type 1 diabetes develops when beta cells in the pancreas that produce insulin are destroyed. Scientists have now found that the pancreas has immature beta cells that might help the pancreas to function again.

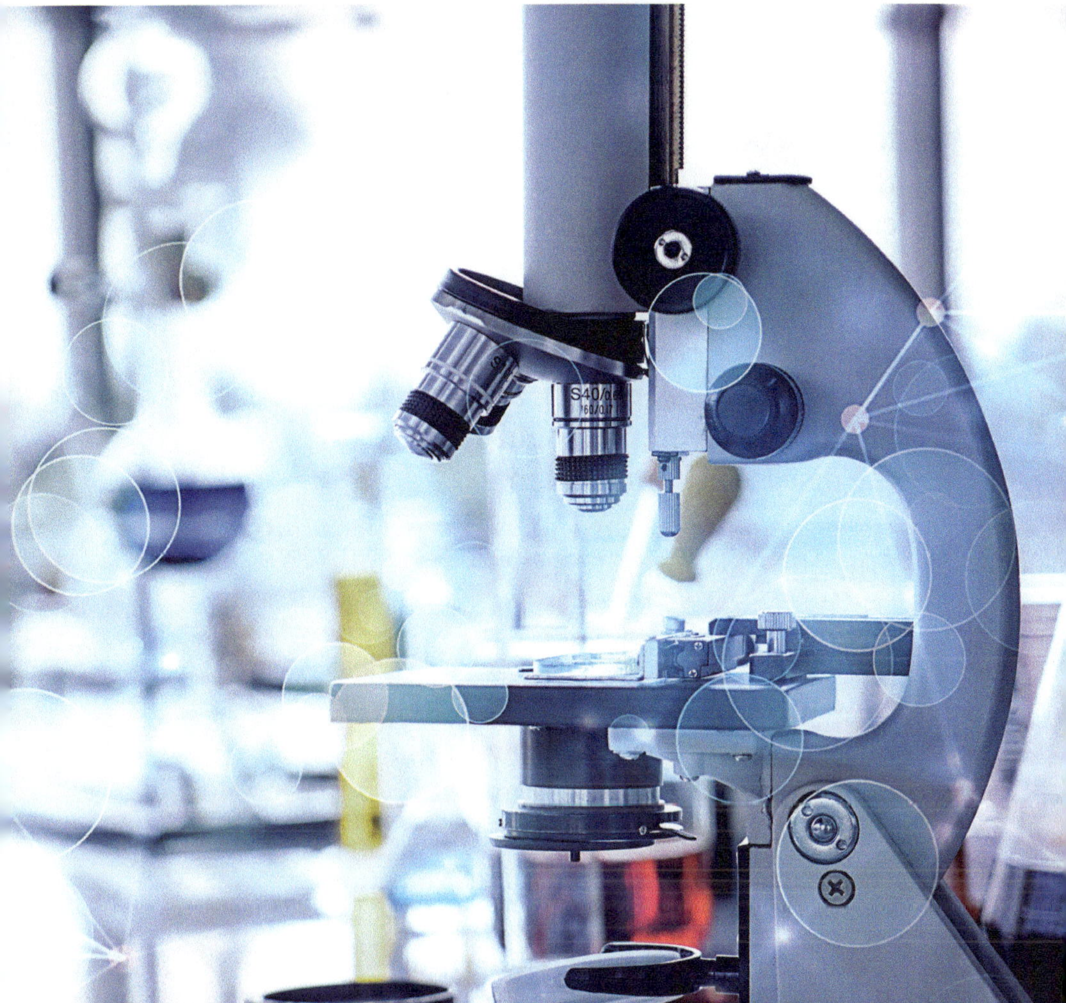

Scientists are constantly working toward finding new and better treatments for diabetes.

To treat type 1 diabetes, researchers are working on small implants that are made from stem cells and produce insulin. Scientists also have made advances in immunotherapy that could prevent type 1 diabetes by making the transplantation of islet cells into the pancreas more successful.

In type 2 diabetes, researchers are working on the causes of insulin resistance. They're devising a therapy for lowering a molecule called ceramides that could reverse insulin resistance. This could make it possible for insulin to work properly again. Also in type 2 diabetes, clinical trials are examining how strict weight management could reverse the disease in some patients.

ADVANCES IN DIABETES TECHNOLOGY

New technology continues to help make it easier for people with diabetes to manage the day-to-day requirements of their condition. A sensor worn on the body gives real-time blood sugar values so diabetics always know whether their numbers are in range. An implantable sensor is being developed that can be worn under the skin for a specific amount of time. Researchers also are working on smart contact lenses that could measure blood glucose as well as deliver drugs to treat diabetic retinopathy.

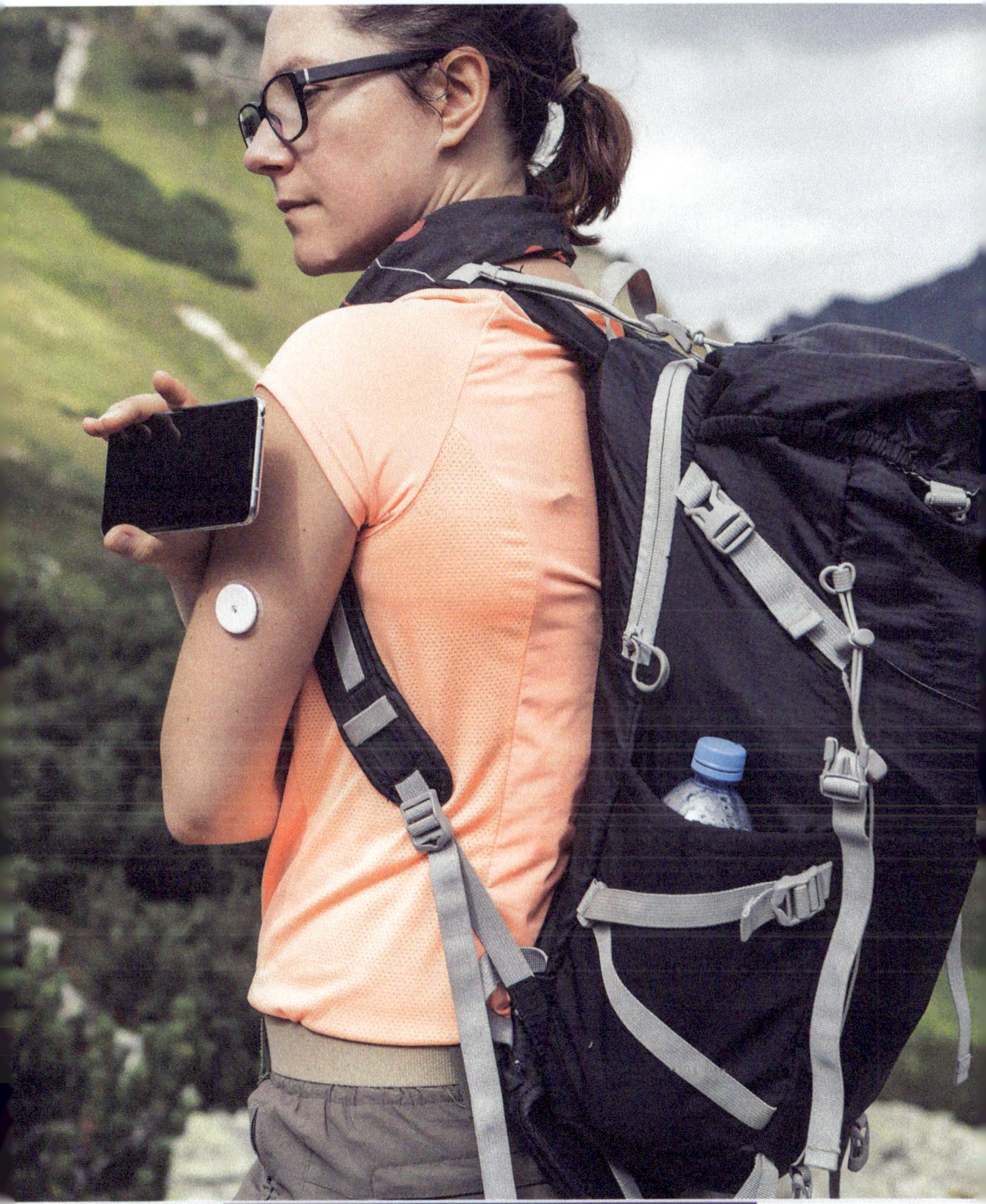

A sensor worn on the body can be read with a device to give a person with diabetes real-time blood glucose values.

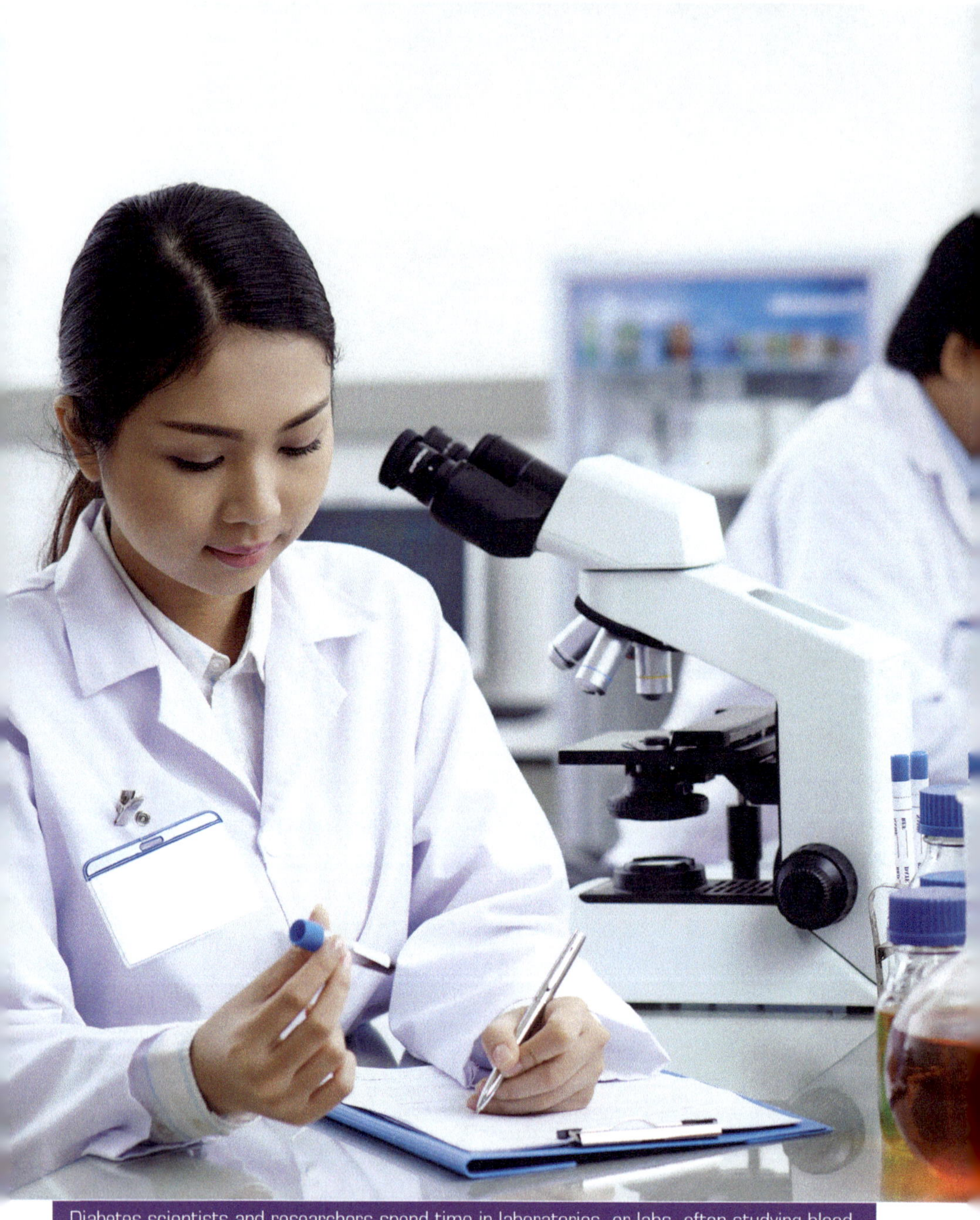

Diabetes scientists and researchers spend time in laboratories, or labs, often studying blood samples from diabetics in an effort to learn more about the condition and find better ways to treat it.

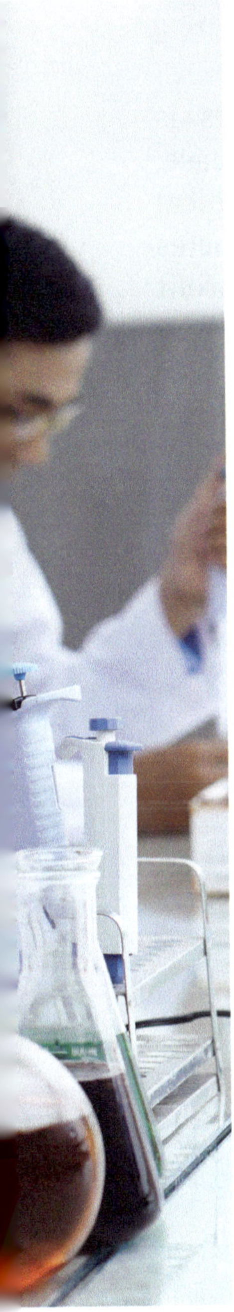

Work continues on what would be a game changer in the treatment of type 1 diabetes. Scientists are seeing how an artificial pancreas system could function automatically with little input required by the wearer.

ADVANCES IN DIABETES MEDICATION

Some commonly used drugs are being investigated to see how they might help in diabetes. A medication used to regulate blood pressure may prevent the autoimmune cause of type 1 diabetes. Immunotherapy treatment is being worked on that might delay the onset of type 1 diabetes in people at risk for developing the disease.

Medications for type 2 diabetes also have evolved to better regulate blood glucose and lower the risk of heart failure in diabetics. Other drugs being developed work to control blood glucose while also protecting the heart and kidneys from the complications of diabetes. Scientists also are working on medication that specifically treats type 2 diabetes in children.

Newer methods of administering glucagon make it easier and, more importantly, faster to treat a low blood sugar emergency. An easier injectable method doesn't require any preparation before using. Another version of glucagon can be given through the nose using a special device.

ADVANCES IN DIABETES AWARENESS

As the cases of diabetes increase, more awareness is needed about what it's like to live with this disease. More funding also is needed to support the clinical trials and research that may one day make diabetes a curable or preventable disease. Many nonprofit organizations work at getting the word out and raising funds.

The advances in medicine and science make living with diabetes easier, along with the possibility of better long-term results. As more options become available, the methods you use today to control your diabetes will change and improve. Research continues on advancing and simplifying the management of diabetes for better outcomes for the millions of people living with diabetes worldwide.

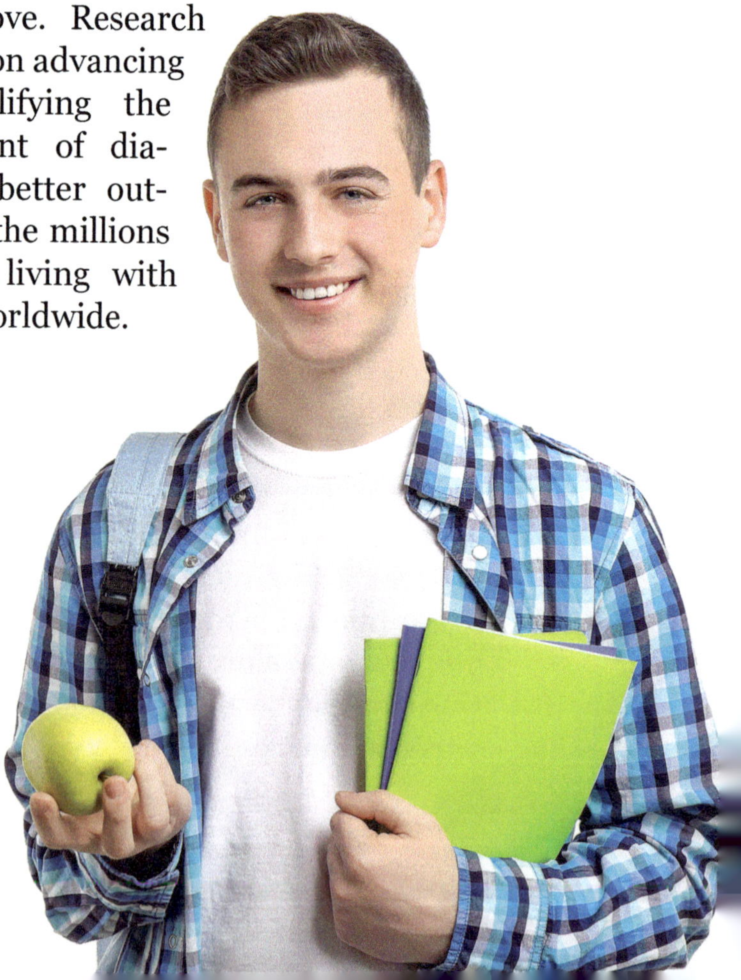

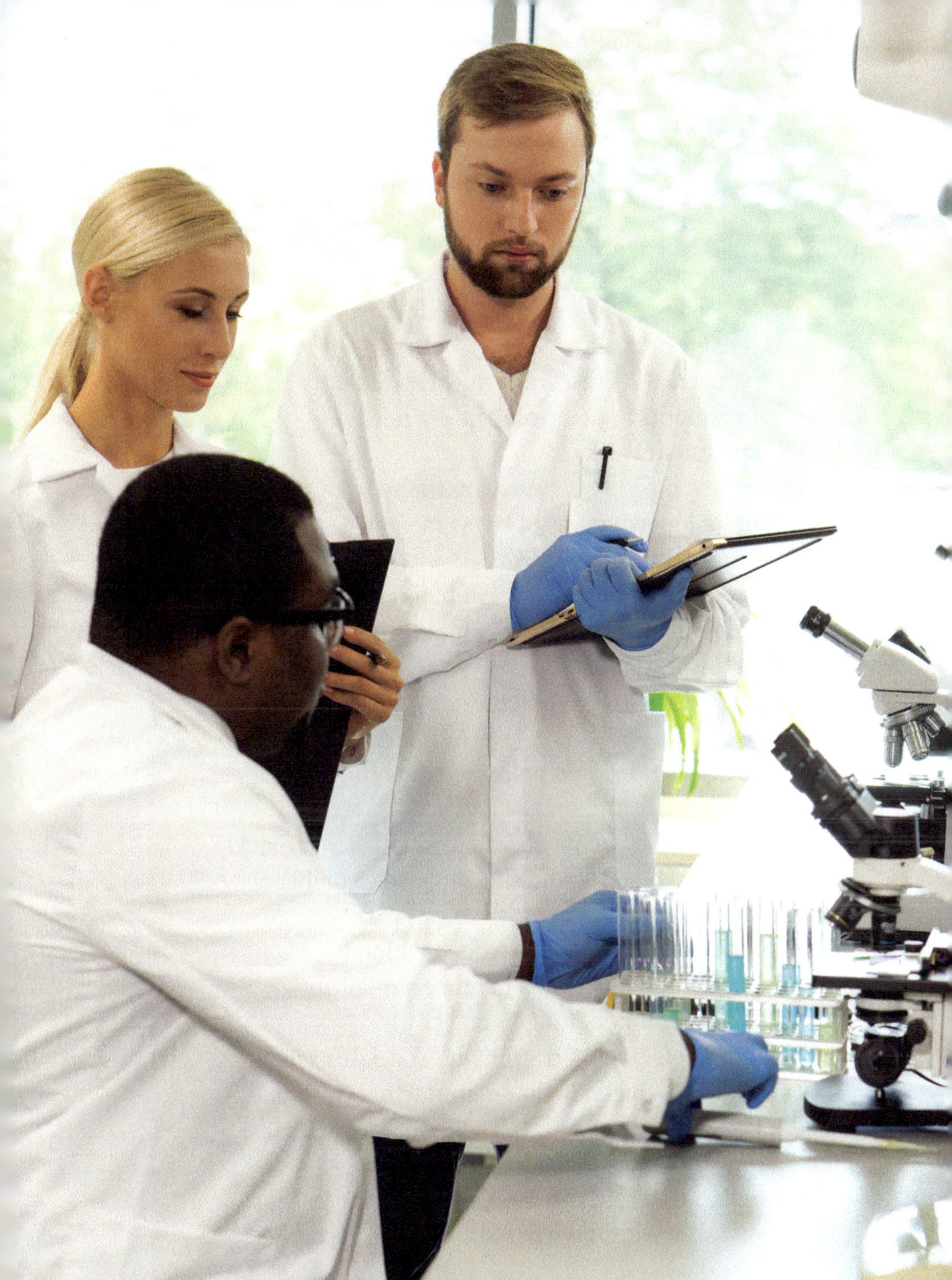

Doctors and scientists continue to research new and less invasive ways for people to manage their diabetes.

GLOSSARY

basal dose: A low, continual dose of insulin.

blood glucose: Also known as blood sugar, it is the amount of sugar found in the bloodstream.

bolus dose: A large dose of insulin taken before meals or snacks.

clinical trial: A research study carried out in patients to determine how a new treatment works.

complex carbohydrate: A carbohydrate made up of longer chains of sugar molecules that takes a longer time to digest.

dawn phenomenon: A high blood sugar value (hyperglycemia) upon waking up in the morning.

diabetes mellitus: A medical term for diabetes.

diabetic ketoacidosis (DKA): A serious complication of diabetes in which the body can't use glucose and breaks down fat instead, resulting in chemicals called ketones that quickly turn the blood acidic and can lead to diabetic coma and death.

dialysis: A process that cleans the blood of waste products in a manner similar to normally functioning kidneys.

endocrinologist: A doctor who specializes in the glands of the body that manufacture hormones.

gestational diabetes: High blood glucose that affects women who are pregnant.

glaucoma: An eye disease marked by increasing pressure within the eyeball that can result in loss of vision.

glucagon: A hormone produced in the pancreas that regulates blood glucose levels.

glucose: A simple sugar that the body converts from food to provide energy to the body.

hormone: A chemical that helps regulate how cells and organs in the body function.

hyperglycemia: A condition when there is too much sugar in the bloodstream.

hypoglycemia: A condition when there isn't enough sugar in the bloodstream.

insulin: A hormone produced by the pancreas that helps move glucose from the bloodstream into the cells where it can be used for energy.

insulin resistance: The ineffective use of insulin by the body.

ketones: The waste product produced when the body breaks down fat to use for energy.

lipodystrophies: Lumps of reorganized fat caused by repeatedly injecting insulin at the same site.

neuropathy: Damage to the nerves, usually in the hands and feet, that causes numbness and weakness.

pancreas: The organ behind the stomach responsible for producing insulin and glucagon.

prediabetes: A condition where blood glucose is higher than normal but isn't yet classified as diabetes.

retinologist: A doctor who specializes in caring for the eyes, especially the retina.

simple carbohydrate: A carbohydrate made up of sugar molecules that takes a shorter time to digest.

FOR MORE INFORMATION

American Diabetes Association (ADA)
2451 Crystal Drive, Suite 900
Alexandria, VA 22202
(800) 342-2383
Website: www.diabetes.org
Facebook: @AmericanDiabetesAssociation
Instagram: @amdiabetesassn
Twitter: @AmDiabetesAssn
The American Diabetes Association is dedicated to improving the lives of people living with diabetes through research and advocating for patients.

Association of Diabetes Care & Education Specialists (ADCES)
125 South Wacker Drive, Suite 600
Chicago, IL 60606
(800) 338-3633
Website: www.diabeteseducator.org/
Facebook and Twitter: @ADCESdiabetes
Proper patient self-management of diabetes is advocated by this association of healthcare professionals.

Beyond Type 1
1001 Laurel Street, Suite B
San Carlos, CA 94070
(650) 924-5959
Website: beyondtype1.org/
Facebook: @BeyondType1
Instagram and Twitter: @beyondtype1

Founded in 2015, this organization brings global awareness to living with a chronic disease through advocacy, education, funding, and resources.

Diabetes Advocacy Alliance
100 College Road West
Princeton, NJ 08540
Website: www.diabetesadvocacyalliance.org/
Twitter: @DiabAdvAlliance
This coalition of patient, professional, and trade groups works toward changing how diabetes is viewed and treated in the United States.

Diabetes Canada
1300-522 University Avenue
Toronto, ON M5G 2R5
Canada
(800) 226-8464
Website: www.diabetes.ca
Facebook, Instagram, and Twitter: @Diabetes-Canada
The primary goal of Diabetes Canada is to help prevent and cure diabetes and to improve the lives of people affected by the disease.

Diabetes Research Institute Foundation (DRI)
200 South Park Road, Suite 100
Hollywood, FL 33021
(800) 321-3437
Website: www.diabetesresearch.org/

Facebook: @DiabetesResearchInstitute
Twitter: @Diabetes_DRI
The Institute focuses its research on finding a cure for diabetes.

Juvenile Diabetes Research Foundation International (JDRF)

200 Vesey Street, 28th Floor
New York, NY 10281
(800) 533-2873
Website: www.jdrf.org
Facebook: @myJDRF
Twitter: @JDRF
The Foundation funds research, advocates for patient access to new therapies, and offers support for people living with Type 1 diabetes worldwide.

National Institute of Diabetes and Digestive and Kidney Diseases (NIDDK)

9000 Rockville Pike
Bethesda, MD 20892
(800) 860-8747
Website: www.niddk.nih.gov
Facebook, Instagram, and Twitter: @NIDDKgov
Founded in 1950, NIDDK research has expanded the knowledge and treatments for diabetes and related diseases.

The diaTribe Foundation
776 Haight Street
San Francisco, CA 94117
(415) 241-9500
Website: diatribe.org/foundation
Facebook and Twitter: @diaTribeNews
Instagram: @diaTribe
This foundation seeks to raise awareness of the growing diabetes epidemic and to advocate for better patient outcomes.

FOR FURTHER READING

Brown, Adam. *Bright Spots and Landmines: The Diabetes Guide I Wish Someone Had Handed Me.* San Francisco: The diaTribe Foundation, 2017.

Colberg, Sheri R, PhD. *The Athlete's Guide to Diabetes.* Champaign, IL: Human Kinetics Publishers, 2019.

Hanas, Ragnar, MD. *Type 1 Diabetes in Children, Adolescents, and Young Adults, Seventh Edition.* Cambridge, MA: Class Health, 2019.

Hergenreter, Valorie. *I'm Still Me, Can't You See? Diabetes Won't Stop Me.* Eugene, OR: Luminare Press, 2016.

McAllister, Patrick. *Highs & Lows of Type 1 Diabetes: The Ultimate Guide for Teens and Young Adults.* New York, NY: Good Books, 2018.

Pelicano, Matt. *Tabouli: The Story of a Heart-Driven Diabetes Alert Dog.* Greenville, SC: April Fool Publishing, 2019.

Ross, Tami A, RDN, LD, CDE, MLDE, FAADE. *What Do I Eat Now? A Guide to Eating Well with Diabetes and Prediabetes.* Arlington, VA: American Diabetes Association, 2020.

Scheiner, Gary, MS, CDCES. *Think Like a Pancreas: A Practical Guide to Managing Diabetes with Insulin, Third Edition*. New York, NY: Hachette Books, 2020.

Warren, Ariel, RDN, CDCES. *Type 1 Diabetes for the Newly Diagnosed: What to Expect, What to Do, How to Thrive*. Emeryville, CA, and New York: Rockridge Press, 2020.

Wilson, Val, MD. *How to Live Well with Diabetes: A Comprehensive Guide to Taking Control of Your Life with Diabetes*. Boston, MA: Little, Brown, and Company, 2019.

INDEX

ABOUT THE AUTHOR

Henrietta Toth has written several nonfiction books for children. She is an editor with 20 years of experience in academic publishing. She has learned a lot by working on books about many different topics. She has learned about diabetes from her father and niece as they manage their diabetes and she dedicates this book to them. She also acknowledges the assistance of Clara Tóth, PhD, in preparing this edition.

CREDITS

Photo Credits: Cover, New Africa/Shutterstock.com; Cover, pp. 1–104 LUMIKK555/Shutterstock.com; Cover, pp. 1–104 Filin84/Shutterstock.com; p. 5 Olga Miltsova/Shutterstock.com; pp. 7, 41 Photographee.eu/Shutterstock.com; p. 8 garagestock/Shutterstock.com; p. 10 Magic mine/Shutterstock.com; p. 13 https://en.wikipedia.org/wiki/File:Areteo_di_Cappadocia.jpg; p. 15 Science Photo Library/Getty Images; p. 17 Jacobs Stock Photography/Photodisc/Getty Images; p. 19 Daisy Daisy/Shutterstock.com; p. 21 Prostock-studio/Shutterstock.com; p. 23 ER Productions Limited/DigitalVision/Getty Images; p. 27 File:C. H. Best and F. G. Banting ca. 1924.png; p. 28 Monkey Business Images/Shutterstock.com; p. 30 Hinterhaus Productions/DigitalVision/Getty Images; pp. 33, 55 fizkes/Shutterstock.com; p. 35 sturti/E+/Getty Images; p. 36 Asia Images Group/Getty Images; p. 38 Ariel Skelley/DigitalVision/Getty Images; p. 43 Andrey_Popov/Shutterstock.com; p. 44 Branimir76/E+/Getty Images; p. 46 Carlo Prearo/EyeEm/Getty Images; p. 49 ljubaphoto/E+/Getty Images; p. 51 Cozine/Shutterstock.com; p. 52 Eva-Katalin/E+/Getty Images; p. 57 Peter Dazeley/The Image Bank/Getty Images; p. 59 Jacek Chabraszewski/Shutterstock.com; p. 61 ER Productions Limited/ DigitalVision/Getty Images; p. 63 Magic mine/Shutterstock.com; p. 65 Elnur/Shutterstock.com; p. 67 Bernd Schwabedissen/EyeEm/Getty Images; p. 68 WilleeCole Photography/Shutterstock.com; p. 70 Portra/DigitalVision/Getty Images; p. 72 cheapbooks/Shutterstock.com; p. 75 BR Photo Addicted/Shutterstock.com; p. 76 Halfpoint/Shutterstock.com; p. 79 monzenmachi/E+/Getty Images; p.81 sturti/E+/Getty Images; p. 82 Branislav Nenin/Shutterstock.com; p. 85 DFree/Shutterstock.com; p. 87 Mongkolchon Akesin/Shutterstock.com; p. 89 Lukasz Pawel Szczepanski/Shutterstock.com; p. 90 Dragon Images/Shutterstock.com; p. 92 Pixel-Shot/Shutterstock.com; p. 93 Maksim Shmeljov/Shutterstock.com.